Teaching in Your Office

For a catalogue of publications available from ACP-ASIM, contact:

Customer Service Center
American College of Physicians–American Society of Internal Medicine
190 N. Independence Mall West
Philadelphia, PA 19106-1572
215-351-2600
800-523-1546, ext. 2600

Visit our Web site at www.acponline.org

Teaching in Your Office

A Guide to Instructing Medical Students and Residents

Patrick C. Alguire, MD, FACP
Director, Education and Career Development
American College of Physicians–American Society of Internal Medicine

Dawn E. DeWitt, MD, MSc, FACP
Assistant Professor of Medicine, University of Washington
Medicine Residency WWAMI Coordinator
UWMC Ambulatory and Wyoming Medicine Clerkship Coordinator
Rural/Underserved Opportunities Program Faculty Liaison

Linda E. Pinsky, MD
Director of Resident Ambulatory Education
Assistant Professor of Medicine
Adjunct Assistant Professor of Medical Education
University of Washington

Gary S. Ferenchick, MD, FACP
Associate Professor of Internal Medicine
Clerkship Director
Michigan State University

AMERICAN COLLEGE OF PHYSICIANS
Philadelphia, Pennsylvania

Manager, Book Publishing: David Myers
Administrator, Book Publishing: Diane McCabe
Production Supervisor: Allan S. Kleinberg
Production Editor: Scott Thomas Hurd
Developmental Editor: Vicki Hoenigke
Editorial Assistant: Alicia Dillihay
Indexer: Dorothy Hoffman
Designer: Kate Nichols

Printed in the United States of America
Composition by Fulcrum Data Services, Inc.
Printing/binding by Versa Press

American College of Physicians (ACP) became an imprint of the American College of Physicians–American Society of Internal Medicine in July 1998.

Library of Congress Cataloging-in-Publication Data

Learners in your office : a guide to teaching medical students and residents / Patrick Alguire . . . [et al.]
  p.; cm.
  Includes bibliographical references and index.
  ISBN 1-930513-07-0
  1. Medicine--Study and teaching (Preceptorship)--United States.
  2. Ambulatory medical care--Study and teaching--United States.
  3. Medicine--Study and teaching (Residency)--United States.
  4. Medical offices. I. Alguire, Patrick C. (Patrick Craig), 1950–
  [DNLM: 1. Education, Medical--methods. 2. Preceptorship--methods.
  3. Teaching--methods. W 20 L4373 2000]
  R837.P74 L43 2000
  610'.71'173--dc21

01 02 03 04 05 / 9 8 7 6 5 4 3 2 1

Contents

Preface

Teaching in Your Office is a resource for physicians interested in improving their skills in office-based teaching. The reason that such a book is needed is evidenced by the very nature of ambulatory teaching. Ambulatory medical education takes place in a fast-paced, chaotic environment in which there is little time for teaching, observation, and feedback. The office practice, in particular, is seen as being able to offer few opportunities for reflection and collaborative learning or teaching (1). Office-based preceptors often believe that they have no occasion to observe others teach and to receive feedback on their own teaching skills. Consequently, preceptors mistakenly consider the opportunity for self-improvement to be limited.

This book intends to help office-based physicians improve their own teaching while maintaining the efficiency of their practice. It is designed to allow busy clinicians to identify and read only those chapters that address their specific needs. In other words, *Teaching in Your Office* does not need to be read cover to cover; rather, it can be read selectively. Additionally, each major topic area in the teaching skills and organizational chapters (Chapters 3 and 4) is summarized for quick review in Appendix A: Quick Tips for Preceptors. Similarly, if you begin reading the summaries first, the page locations of any associated text are indicated after the summary headings.

The following paragraphs describe each of the major sections and who would benefit from reading them.

Making an Informed Decision About Precepting (Chapter 1)

This chapter is for physicians who have never taught in their offices and want to know why they should teach, what teaching entails, and its potential costs and benefits. This section also describes the "prerequisites" for office-based teaching and where to turn for help in improving teaching skills.

The Curriculum (Chapter 2)

This chapter describes what the student or resident is expected to accomplish when participating in an office-based teaching experience. It is useful for 1) physicians who teach, but who have not been told *what* to teach; and 2) clinicians who have been asked to help plan an office-based curriculum.

Getting Ready To Teach (Chapter 3)

This chapter describes how to 1) prepare the office and staff for teaching, 2) conduct learner orientation, and 3) schedule patients when a learner is present. It also addresses how to document a patient visit for billing purposes when a learner has participated in patient care. This section will be particularly helpful for new teachers or teachers trying to improve their efficiency.

Teaching Skills and Organizational Techniques for Office-Based Teaching (Chapter 4)

This chapter provides a definition of meaningful patient responsibility, describes the characteristics of effective teachers, and provides tips on how to help learners organize their visit with the patient. Novices and experienced teachers will benefit from this chapter.

Case-Based Learning (Chapter 5)

This chapter defines case-based learning and provides descriptions of 1) several case-based learning models for office-based teaching, 2) the pitfalls of case-based learning, and 3) how to conclude the day. All preceptors will benefit from reading this section.

Ways to Be More Efficient When Teaching (Chapter 6)

This chapter presents tips on how to teach efficiently (getting more done in less time) yet effectively. The contents of this section were set aside specifically for preceptors wishing to minimize the effect of office-based teaching on productivity or the length of their day; however, it contains useful teaching suggestions for all preceptors, regardless of concerns about efficiency.

Learner Feedback and Evaluation (Chapter 7)

This section describes how to give effective feedback to learners, evaluate a learner, and use a simple yet valid evaluation model. This section concludes with advice on how to avoid common evaluation errors and how to conduct the final evaluation session. All preceptors should read the sections on feedback, whereas preceptors who must provide a formal evaluation of the learner to the sponsoring institution should review the section on evaluation.

Preceptor Evaluation and Teaching Improvement (Chapter 8)

This chapter provides 1) information on how preceptors are evaluated by their learners, 2) examples of how this information is used by the sponsoring institution, and 3) tips on how to continue the process of improving teaching skills.

Tips, Tools, and Resources (Appendices A, B, and C)

Collected in the back of the book are summaries of the major points described in the text, useful data-collection and organizational tools, and resources intended to make the job of teaching easier and more efficient. Some experienced teachers may prefer to read only this section as a "refresher," but most preceptors will find the material in this section helpful both as a summary and as a source of practical teaching aids.

Patrick C. Alguire, MD

1

Making an Informed
Decision About Precepting

The information provided in this chapter is intended to help physicians not currently involved in office-based teaching make an appropriate decision about participation. This section provides background information about office-based teaching (also called community-based teaching), including why it is needed, its contributions and effectiveness, patient satisfaction, and preceptor costs and benefits.

❖ What Is Community-Based Teaching?

Community-based teaching is a return to the historical roots of medical education—the one-on-one teaching of students and residents by practitioners in an office setting. Community-based teachers are most frequently described as teaching physicians who do not have full-time academic appointments; however, exceptions to this rule are common, and many full-time academic physicians who deliver care in (nonhospital) office settings are considered community-based teachers. Some community-based teachers receive a financial stipend for their participation, but many do not. What these groups have in common is the delivery of comprehensive, primary, or subspecialty care in an ambulatory setting to patients who recognize the practitioner as their personal physician. Community-based teaching establishes an environment of "educational intimacy," consisting of one teacher, one learner, and one patient—a place where role modeling, assessment, feedback, and evaluation are maximized for the benefit of the learner (1).

❖ Why Is Community-Based Teaching Needed?

Teaching institutions need community-based practitioners who are willing to teach in their offices. Decreasing numbers of inpatients and the growing mismatch between the educational content and clinical practice of medicine have resulted in a greater emphasis on ambulatory training. Ambulatory settings provide the best opportunity to learn about common office-based problems, chronic disease management, screening, health maintenance, doctor-patient relationships, and some psychosocial aspects of care (2,3). However, not all ambulatory settings are equal. The traditional ambulatory environment is the academic medical center or the hospital-based clinic. In this setting, a single faculty member may supervise three to five learners caring for patients who may not recognize the supervising faculty as their "personal physician." In contrast, the practitioner's office can provide an outstanding educational environment with one-to-one mentoring. Also, the close relationships that develop between physicians and learners provide an opportunity for role modeling that cannot be reproduced in other settings.

The growth of community-based teaching is most impressive and is rapidly becoming the standard for medical student and resident education. For example, in 1984, office assignments for internal medicine residents were offered by only 7% of residency programs (4); in 1998, over 90% exposed at least some of their residents to community-based teaching and nearly half of these exposed more than 80% of their residents to an office setting. For those programs offering community-based training, such exposure accounted for more than 10% training time for upper-level residents (Unpublished data, American College of Physicians–American Society of Internal Medicine [ACP-ASIM]).

However, this success has created problems. Office-based preceptors are a scarce commodity. Nearly half of clerkship administrators at medical schools and approximately two thirds of residency-program directors indicate that the current amount of ambulatory training time is insufficient to meet their curricular needs. The barrier that prevents the medical schools and residency programs from meeting their goals is the inadequate number of training sites and preceptors (5). The process of recruiting qualified preceptors is a difficult one, and it may be getting harder (6). A preponderance of schools report that preceptors are less likely to volunteer because of economic pressures in their offices that force them to become more efficient. Other reasons for diminishing numbers include 1) more competition between schools and residency programs for preceptors, and 2) the demand for preceptors exceeding the supply (6). Thus, there is an urgent need to attract more physicians to community-based teaching programs to bolster medical school and residency programs.

❖ How Good Is the Training in Community Offices?

Office-based teaching offers certain educational experiences that are more representative of "real world" medicine compared with the traditional hospital-based clinic. Students in community-based settings see more patients, are exposed to a wider variety of patient problems, provide more acute care, evaluate more patients in the emergency department, and perform more procedures than students assigned to traditional hospital-based clinics. Furthermore, compared with students in traditional clinic settings, students in community-settings are more likely to be supervised closely, to see patients in follow-up, to discuss the patient's case with a preceptor, to witness the preceptor delivering care, and to rate their experiences highly (3,7–10).

There are concerns that students assigned to ambulatory settings away from the academic medical center will not master the required medical content. Data to support or refute this point of view are difficult to collect. The published studies to date show no evidence of decreased mastery of core content when students are assigned on a part-time basis to community offices compared with students who receive all of their training at academic medical centers. Although most of these studies were not randomized—which decreases their validity—the results of these nonrandomized studies are encouraging. Compared with students at academic medical centers (including hospital-based ambulatory clinics), students assigned on a part-time basis to community offices have similar scores on end-of-rotation evaluation exercises, including oral examinations, practical clinical examinations, and the National Board of Medical Examiners subject examination. Furthermore, students spending part of their training time in a practitioner's office have similar clerkship grades and number of honors grades compared with students who receive all of their training at the academic medical center (7,11). On the other hand, students trained in part-time office settings may have improved skills in clinical diagnosis, laboratory interpretation, doctor-patient relationships, and communication skills compared with their peers trained entirely in the academic medical center (3,11–14).

Fears that the office-based experience does not sufficiently involve students in patient care also seem to be unfounded. Students report that they are just as involved in patient care as when they were in the hospital, i.e., they have adequate supervision, have sufficient learning time, see a wider variety of patients and problems, and perform minimal "scut" work (12). Finally, residents rate their quality of supervision in private offices as being better than what they experienced in institutional clinics or health-maintenance organizations (HMOs) (15).

In summary, the available data suggest that office-based training seems more enjoyable, varied, active, and supervised than traditional training.

❖ What Do Community-Based Practitioners Have To Offer Learners?

Many physicians are reluctant to participate in community-based teaching because they believe they lack the time and talent to "teach." In this context, teaching is mistakenly translated by community physicians as providing "lectures." In fact, this is not what learners, medical schools, and residency programs want from preceptors; they want exposure to practical skills. In this light, most community-based physicians *can* teach efficiently and effectively. For example, in one study, students were asked to identify critical learning events that took place in office-based settings. Typically, these important teaching moments lasted less than five minutes, focused on problems (rather than on an abstract review of a topic), and had a practical outcome. The single most important learning event identified by students was observing an experienced physician interacting with a patient. This is not to suggest that the entire experience should be observational. On the contrary, students and residents crave the opportunity to deliver independent care (i.e., first seeing the patient alone, then with the preceptor), but the opportunity to witness an expert deal with a difficult problem is highly valued. Other highly rated learning events include improving communication and clinical skills (12,16). These are important abilities that preceptors have in abundance, and they require little in the way of preparation to be presented effectively to the learner.

The take-home message to office-based preceptors is that a student who participates in an office-based experience values learning the process of care as much as, or possibly more than, mastering core content. Students and residents crave the real-world experience of caring for patients, which office-based practitioners can provide.

❖ How Do Learners Rate the Community Experience and Preceptors?

Students and residents value their time with community preceptors and recognize the unique contributions the office-based experience brings to their training. Student evaluations of volunteer preceptors are rated as highly as full-time faculty (17), but community faculty are rated higher in showing interest (10). When students were asked to compare their community-based experience with other clerkships, the office experience was seen as contributing most to their acquisition of improved clinical and communication skills and improved awareness of issues relating to cost-effectiveness. Comparing their community-based experiences with traditional clerkship rotations, students reported learning as much about disease pattern recognition and the ability to generate a differential diagnosis and actually learned *more* about evaluating "hidden agenda" items and about managing chronic medical and psychosocial problems (12,16,18).

❖ What Are the Concerns of Practitioners Involved in Community-Based Teaching?

Practitioners involved in office-based teaching frequently voice concerns over potential costs and time required for teaching (2,19). Other concerns include 1) poor matching of student with preceptor; 2) dealing with potential teacher-learner conflicts, poorly motivated learners, and inappropriate learner behavior; and 3) the effect of office teaching on patient satisfaction (20). Preceptors are concerned about their ability to provide a good educational experience for the learner and their lack of resources (e.g., textbooks, computers) to support teaching (20). Preceptors are uncomfortable giving feedback to students, particularly if it is negative, and preceptors want to be assured that the institution will cover the learner's malpractice insurance, which it will. The following paragraphs address these important concerns and provide physicians with the necessary information to help them decide whether or not they want to be an office-based preceptor.

❖ What Are Some of the Costs Associated with Community-Based Teaching?

The two most commonly cited costs of office-based teaching are preceptor time and lost billings. Most studies involving students show an increase in the workday of 45 minutes to an hour for each half-day teaching session (19,21). Results of studies assessing productivity vary from showing no loss of productivity or revenue (but a longer workday) to seeing one less patient each half-day session, corresponding to reduced charges of $55 to $60 (21–26). In one study, however, two thirds of physicians reported no loss of income (19). The presence of a student does not seem to be associated with increased "hidden costs" (e.g., more laboratory tests, prescriptions, or referrals to other physicians), an important consideration in a "managed" health care system (27).

Other studies have documented that the time actually spent in direct contact with a student is just over three hours for each half-day session, considerably more than the time documented for inpatient teaching (28). Approximately 45 minutes to an hour of the contact time is spent alone with the student; the balance is with the student and patient (25,28). Studies have not been reported for residents participating in office-based teaching; however, it is likely that the results would be similar. Although residents are more clinically capable, most practitioners see residents' patients (briefly) to maintain the doctor-patient relationship and to justify billing.

❖ What Are the Practitioner Benefits of Community-Based Teaching?

Community preceptors repeatedly report that precepting makes them enjoy clinical practice more (19,25,29,30). Most preceptors report a fulfilling sense of "giving something back" to medicine (31). Others have commented on a decreased sense of professional isolation and the rewards of sharing knowledge and a vision of the

specialty with the learner (30). Keeping up with the medical literature and reviewing basic sciences and clinical skills also are frequently reported as benefits of community-based teaching
(25,30,31). Some physicians and institutions use precepting as a
method to recruit newly graduated residents as employees or partners (19,32). There is even a suggestion that office-based education
results in increased time spent in patient education, a value-added
benefit of teaching that is reaped by patients (29). One potential
economic windfall is a higher capitation rate for participating physicians negotiated in their behalf by the training institution. A 1%
increase in the capitation rate has been negotiated by medical
schools, which is a tangible reward despite its tendency to be a
rather small sum of money (32). This strategy can be employed by
most teaching institutions for their office preceptors.

❖ What Are the Most Commonly Offered Rewards for Community-Based Teaching?

Most preceptors are rewarded for their participation in office-based
teaching programs, but typically the reward is not financial. Just
over half of medical schools provide clinical appointments to volunteer faculty, but only 15% provide a financial stipend (8,22). Some
state legislatures, including those of Georgia, Alabama, and Texas,
provide direct compensation to office-based preceptors for certain
teaching programs.

Although it is likely that practitioners would appreciate financial
reimbursement for their efforts, most acknowledge that institutions
cannot begin to pay what their teaching is worth. Nevertheless, practitioners are consistent in their desire to have their contribution rec-
ognized in some meaningful way (8,21,22,30,33). The value of the
reward to the practitioner differs according to the practice type and
location (33). (*See the section entitled "Commonly Offered Rewards for
Precepting" on page 136 for a more detailed description.*)

❖ What Do Learners Want from a Community-Based Teaching Experience?

Again, the message from the learners is consistent and clear: they want the opportunity to practice patient management, basic data collection, and interpretation skills on the wide variety of patients typically seen in the office setting. They desire feedback on their performance and a role model to emulate. To students, the preceptor's characteristics are the most important factor defining a successful office-based experience; of these, the most highly rated is the preceptor's ability to promote student independence (34). Most often this is accomplished by giving the student increasing patient care responsibility. Other highly favored characteristics include the preceptor's willingness to allow the student 1) to practice technical and problem-solving skills, 2) to show enthusiasm and interest in patients, and 3) to be actively involved in the learning process. The willingness of a preceptor to act as a mentor and to advise the student is also highly valued (12,16,34).

Although the characteristics of the office itself are important to learners, they are secondary to preceptor characteristics. Valued office characteristics include having many different preceptors available, a variety of patient problems, and a range of patient ages (34).

The areas that provide the most difficulty for students are learning to work within the time constraints of the office setting, performing a focused examination, and learning to rely on data-gathering skills and problem-solving abilities rather than on imaging and laboratory tests (35). Preceptors, by virtue of their everyday experience, can provide valuable tips and direction to help learners develop these skill sets. Residents value the opportunity to discuss differential diagnosis and management issues, and they appreciate close supervision, feedback, and the opportunity to practice and improve clinical and procedural skills (36).

❖ How Do Patients React to Office-Based Teaching?

One reason physicians may not participate in office-based teaching is their concerns about quality of care and patient satisfaction when a learner is in the office (5). To address these concerns, studies have been performed in both staff-model HMOs and traditional office practices. In the HMO setting, over 90% of the participating physicians and their patients indicated that quality of care and patient satisfaction were unaffected by the presence of students (25). Similar results can be found in surveys of physicians in private practice and by questioning their patients directly (27). Many patients report enjoying the extra attention they receive from the learner and are impressed that their personal physician is involved in training students and residents (37). Negative reactions to students are uncommon even around issues of repeating parts of the examination performed by the student, discussing personal issues in front of a student, or extending the length of the visit (37). Despite the rarity of negative experiences, it remains the prerogative of the patient to decline participation in office-based teaching, and consent always should be obtained before involving a student or resident in their care.

❖ What Are the Prerequisites for Precepting?

Most institutions that need community-based preceptors do not require previous teaching experience as a pre-requisite. In fact, few full-time academic faculty have ever been taught how to teach. Nevertheless, faculty-development programs can be a helpful resource to improve teaching effectiveness and are recommended. In the interim, most community physicians can provide useful educational experiences to learners without formal training in teaching. Keep in mind that what most learners want out of the experience is the opportunity to observe problems common to the ambulatory setting and then to practice treating them. They also desire feedback on their performance. Learners in the ambulatory setting are less interested in lectures and more interested in the "how to" process. Learners crave "real world" experiences with role models that care for patients. It is also important to understand that learners don't want a "shadowing" experience, i.e., following a preceptor from patient to patient simply observing the care that is given. Essentially, learners want meaningful and independent responsibility. Initially, this means having opportunities to see the patient alone. After this step, there are many teaching strategies that detail how to teach and provide care in ways that are efficient and satisfying to both the learner and the patient (*see Chapter 5*).

❖ Are There Courses To Improve Your Teaching?

For those interested in improving their teaching skills, this book helps lay a foundation; however, as with any learning situation, being observed and receiving feedback is probably the most effective method to improve your teaching. Many medical schools and residency programs provide workshops designed to improve teaching, and they will be happy to involve you. Some teaching workshops are offered at national meetings, such as ACP-ASIM's Annual Session.

Due to their timing, duration, or location, faculty-development workshops may not be a feasible option for all physicians. To meet the needs of these preceptors, some teaching programs have put their faculty-development programs on the Internet or on CD-ROM, or they have created instructional videotapes and companion texts. Most of these programs are free or available for a modest price. For a listing of available faculty-development workshops or resources near you, call the Community-Based Teaching Program at ACP-ASIM (800-523-1546, ext. 2588) or visit the ACP-ASIM Web site at http//:www.acponline.org/cme/cbt (*see also Appendix C*).

REFERENCES

1. **Irby DM.** Teaching and learning in ambulatory care settings: a thematic review of the literature. *Acad Med.* 1995;70:898–931.
2. **Woolliscroft JO, Schwenk TL.** Teaching and learning in the ambulatory setting. *Acad Med.* 1989;64:644–8.

3. **Butterfield PS, Libertin AG.** Learning outcomes of an ambulatory care rotation in internal medicine for junior medical students. *J Gen Intern Med.* 1993;8:189–92.

4. **Napodano RJ, Schuster BL, Krackov SK, et al.** Use of private offices in education of residents in internal medicine. *Arch Intern Med.* 1984;144:303–5.

5. **Levinsky NG.** A survey of changes in the proportions of ambulatory training in internal medicine and residencies from 1986–1987 and from 1996–1997. *Acad Med.* 1998;73:1114–5.

6. **Barzansky B, Jonas HS, Etzel SI.** Educational programs in U.S. medical schools, 1998–1999. *JAMA.* 1999;282:840–6.

7. **Osborn LM, Sargent JR, Williams SD.** Effects of time-in-clinic setting, and faculty supervision on the continuity clinic experience. *Pediatrics.* 1993;91:1089–93.

8. **Usatine RP, Lin K.** Free Internet access for community physicians. *Acad Med.* 1999;74:204–5.

9. **Greer T, Schneeweiss R, Baldwin LM.** A comparison of student clerkship experiences in community practices and residency-based clinics. *Fam Med.* 1993;25:322–6.

10. **Schwiebert LP, Ramsey CNJ, Davis A.** Comparison of volunteer and full-time faculty performance in a required third-year medicine clerkship. *Teach Learn Med.* 1992;4:225–32.

11. **Pangaro L, Gibson K, Russell W, et al.** A prospective randomized trial of a six-week ambulatory medicine rotation. *Acad Med.* 1995;70:537–41.

12. **Prislin MD, Feighny KM, Stearns JA, et al.** What students say about learning and teaching in longitudinal ambulatory primary care clerkships: a multi-institutional study. *Acad Med.* 1998;73:680–7.

13. **Grum CM, Case SM, Swanson DB, Woolliscroft JO.** Identifying the trees in the forest: characteristics of students who demonstrate disparity between knowledge and diagnostic pattern recognition skills. *Acad Med.* 1994;10(Suppl):S66–8.

14. **Papadakis M, Kagawa MK.** A randomized controlled pilot study of placing third-year medical clerks in a continuity clinic. *Acad Med.* 1993;68:845–7.

15. **Swing SR, Vasilias J.** Internal medicine residency education in ambulatory settings. *Acad Med.* 1997;72:988–96.

16. **Epstein RM, Cole DR, Gawinski BA, et al.** How students learn from community-based preceptors. *Arch Fam Med.* 1998;7:149–54.

17. **Irby DM, Gillmore GM, Ramsey PG.** Factors affecting ratings of clinical teachers by medical students and residents. *J Med Educ.* 1987;62:1–7.

18. **Packman CH, Krackov SK, Groff GD, Cohen J.** The Rochester practice-based experience: an experiment in medical education. *Arch Intern Med.* 1994;154:1253–60.

19. **Vinson DC, Paden C.** The effect of teaching medical students on private practitioner's workloads. *Acad Med.* 1994;69:237–8.

20. **Kollisch DO, Frasier PY, Slatt L, Storaasli M.** Community preceptors' views of a required third-year family medicine clerkship. *Arch Fam Med.* 1997;6:25–8.

21. **Levy BT, Gjerde CL, Albrecht LA.** The effects of precepting on and the support desired by community-based preceptors in Iowa. *Acad Med.* 1997;72:382–4.

22. **Vinson DC, Paden C, Devera-Sales A, et al.** Teaching medical students in community-based practices: a national survey of generalist physicians. *J Fam Prac.* 1997;45:487–94.

23. **Fields SA, Toffler WL, Bledsoe NM.** Impact of the presence of a third-year medical student on gross charges and patient volumes in 22 rural community practices. *Acad Med.* 1994;69(Suppl 10):S87–9.

24. **Kearl GW, Mainous AG.** Physicians' productivity and teaching responsibilities. *Acad Med.* 1993;68:166–7.

25. **Kirz HL, Larsen C.** Costs and benefits of medical student training to a health maintenance organization. *JAMA.* 1986;256:734–9.

26. **Foley R, Yonke A, Smith J, et al.** Recruiting and retaining volunteer community preceptors. *Acad Med.* 1996;71:460–3.

27. **Frank SH, Stange KC, Langa D, Workings M.** Direct observation of community-based ambulatory encounters involving medical students. *JAMA.* 1997;278:712–6.

28. **Ricer RE, Van Horne A, Filak AT.** Costs of preceptors' time spent teaching during a third-year family medicine outpatient rotation. *Acad Med.* 1997;72:547–51.

29. **Grayson MS, Klein M, Lugo J, Visintainer P.** Benefits and costs to community-based physicians teaching primary care to medical students. *J Gen Intern Med.* 1998;13:485–8.

30. **Fulkerson PK, Wang-Cheng R.** Community-based faculty: motivations and rewards. *Fam Med.* 1997;29:105–7.

31. **Dodson MC.** Should private practitioners be paid for teaching? *Acad Med.* 1998;73:222.

32. **Grayson MS, Newton DA, Klein M, Irons T.** Promoting institutional change to encourage primary care: experiences at New York Medical College and East Carolina University School of Medicine. *Acad Med.* 1999;74(Suppl):S9–15.

33. **Langlois JP.** Support of community-preceptors: What do they need? *Fam Med.* 1995;27:641–5.

34. **Biddle WB, Riesenberg LA, Dacy PA.** Medical student's perceptions of desirable characteristics of primary care teaching sites. *Fam Med.* 1996;28:629–33.

35. **Feltovich J, Mast TA, Soler NG.** Teaching medical students in ambulatory settings in departments of internal medicine. *Acad Med.* 1989;64:36–41.

36. **O'Mallery PG, Kroenke K, Ritter J, et al.** What learners and teachers value most in ambulatory educational encounters: a prospective, qualitative study. *Acad Med.* 1999;74:186–91.

37. **Devera-Sales A, Paden C, Vinson DC.** What do family medicine patients think about medical students' participation in their health care? *Acad Med.* 1999;74:550–2.

2

The Curriculum

❖ **What Are Reasonable Teaching Goals for Community-Based Teaching?**

Community-based teaching sites have been used successfully to teach a wide variety of medical skills, including physical diagnosis, patient interviewing, patient education and counseling, ethics, and subspecialty medicine. However, most medical schools and residency programs use internal medicine, family medicine, and pediatric offices to teach the principles of primary care. The box on page 16 highlights the areas that might be addressed during an office-based teaching experience (1,2).

Observing the natural history of disease usually requires a long-term commitment to a continuity of experience, but it also can be accomplished by observing many patients with the same disease at different stages of severity. The office experience also allows the learner to experience the effect that diseases have on their patients and families. Community-based teaching provides the opportunity for students and residents to learn about practice man-

Cognitive

- ▶ Observing the natural or treated history of disease
- ▶ Understanding the social, financial, and ethical aspects of medical practice

Clinical Problem Solving

- ▶ Learning clinical problem solving
- ▶ Understanding the limits of one's knowledge
- ▶ Sources of information gathering

Knowing When To Refer

Attitudinal and Relationship Skills

- ▶ Developing appropriate professional expectations and attitudes about chronic disease
- ▶ Improving patient communication and negotiation skills
- ▶ Developing strong teacher-student relationships

agement, including financial and reimbursement issues, team care, developing collaborative relationships between patients and health care providers, and the role of preventive care. Office practice is particularly well suited for teaching patient communication and negotiation skills. Not unexpectedly, the office provides an excellent opportunity to learn how to treat common medical problems efficiently and effectively. Finally, the office provides an ideal venue for the teacher to observe the learner's strengths and weaknesses closely, to provide detailed feedback, and to model important behaviors effectively.

Institutions that sponsor office-based teaching will provide, or should be encouraged to provide, their learning objectives and goals to the preceptor. These should explicitly spell out the expectations for the office experience and provide benchmarks for providing feedback and evaluation of the the goals and objectives attained by the learner. However, sometimes institutional goals and objectives are voluminous and overwhelming for preceptors. (*See the section entitled "The*

RIME Evaluation Framework" on page 83 for an alternative set of simple but practical learning expectations.)

Finally, you should encourage students and residents to develop their own learning plans and goals at the beginning of the experience, with the expectation that they will be more pertinent and therefore more effective.

REFERENCES

1. **Woolliscroft JO, Schwenk TL.** Teaching and learning in the ambulatory setting. *Acad Med.* 1989;64:644–48.
2. **Wilkerson L, Armstrong E, Lesky L.** Faculty development for ambulatory teaching. *J Gen Intern Med.* 1990;5(Suppl):S44–53.

3

Getting Ready To Teach

❖ Before the Learner Arrives

A well-designed orientation can ease a learner's transition into the office-based practice. Ideally, before the learner's arrival in your office, the training program will provide a general orientation to the experience (*see "Before the Learner Arrives Preparatory Checklist" on page 94*). The *institution's* orientation for the student will probably include the following items:

- Course syllabus with rotation goals and objectives
- Description of the learner's role in the office
- Outline of the expected teaching and learning activities
- Performance-evaluation criteria
- Recommended readings and resources
- Office-chart organization and techniques for efficient review
- Dictation (only occasionally) and charting skills
- Prescription writing
- Clinic etiquette

Approximately a week in advance of the learner's arrival, review the information you have about the learner and the program. The medical school or residency program should provide you with basic information on the learner. Inquire about this material during your orientation to the educational program. Insist that it arrive far enough in advance to allow you sufficient time to plan the experience. Review the institution's educational goals and objectives. Make sure they are compatible with what you can provide. If you have any questions, clarify them with the sponsoring institution before the learner arrives. Determine what materials and orientation the learner received before coming to the office. If you have additional material about your office that the learner needs, ask the institution to forward them to the learner. For example, you may want the learner to know in advance about dress codes, parking, personal use of the telephone, office hours, days off, and after-hours responsibilities.

Clarify with the institution exactly when the learner will be in the office and any anticipated deviations from the schedule. Establish the process and responsibility for notifying the office if the learner cannot make the scheduled experience due to illness or other unavoidable delay. Determine how easily you can notify the learner if *you* are unexpectedly unavailable. Have the institution give you a reliable phone number of their contact person in case other problems arise. Such problems might include failure of the learner to arrive when expected, a sudden change in the office schedule, or not having the necessary administration forms.

Several days in advance of the learner's arrival, remind your office staff and partners of the start date. Distribute a copy of the learner's application or personal information and schedule. If you haven't already done so, take the time to brief the office staff fully on the learner's participation and duties, including learning experiences that may involve them and their areas of responsibility. Review with the receptionist how they will inform patients about the learner in the office and their role in patient care. Listen to the receptionist practice the presentation to make sure it is offered in a positive and affirmative fashion. Experience has shown that this initial introduction can "make or break" the experience. If your teaching plan includes the learner seeing same-day work in patients, coach the receptionist or nurse making these appointments to deliver the message in a way that supports your teaching effort.

Determine where the learner will park and locate a space in the office for the learner to work and study. Equip the space as necessary with references, note pads, writing utensils, and access to telephone and computer. It is not expected that a learner will have their own telephone and computer, but they should be able to share these tools with others and have reliable accessibility. You may wish to gather all of the office forms that the learner will use in one place, and you or one of your staff should describe when and how to use them. Review with the staff what their roles will be in the learner's orientation. It may be useful to have each member write out their names, location in the office, and a several-sentence description of their responsibilities. Compile this for the learner and save it for use by subsequent learners in the office.

Block out time on your schedule for a learner orientation. On that day, have the learner arrive early or have him or her come the day before. Experience has shown that a minimum of 30 minutes is necessary for a meaningful orientation. Take time to write down what you will cover. Save this to use with other learners and add to it as experience with different learners identifies other orientation needs.

Finally, to be efficient and to maximize your enjoyment, identify at least two examination rooms, one each for yourself and the learner. This will enable the two of you to see different patients simultaneously. Before the learner arrives, make the decision about whether he or she will write or dictate their chart notes (if this is even an option in your office). If you wish the learner to dictate, be prepared to give instruction on how the dictation system works and how you would like it done. Write these instructions down and save them in your orientation file for future use.

❖ When the Learner Arrives

Learning About Each Other

The first meeting with a new student or resident should address mutual expectations (1). You should allow approximately 30 minutes on the first day to greet the learner and share information. Begin with a personal orientation by telling the learner about yourself and your practice, why you chose your specialty, and the rewards it has given you. Then ask some questions about the learner, such as where he or she is from, his or her reasons for entering medicine, and his or her career goals (see "When the Learner Arrives Orientation Checklist" on page 96).

Previous Experiences

Next, follow up with an educational orientation. For example, what were the learner's previous rotations, clerkships, ambulatory experiences, and patient care responsibilities? A useful tool to collect this information is the "Clinical Skills Inventory" (see page 114). This is a simple list of previous learning experiences completed by the learner before beginning the office-based experience. This tool quickly outlines learning needs and can be used to plan the educational content of the experience.

Expectations

This is also a good time to review the institution's expectations with the learner and his or her own goals for the experience. One strategy to accomplish both tasks is developing a learner contract (see "Learner Contract" on page 116). A learner contract outlines the learner's and your expectations for the experience and serves as a guide for your final evaluation of the learner. More simply, a learner contract is a statement of intent or purpose that is described in observable and measurable terms. Examples include the following:

- Performance expected of the learner, preceptor, or both
- Conditions necessary to perform as expected
- Realistic criteria for successful completion of the learning goals (what, where, when, and how)

Consequences of Achieving or Not Achieving Learning Goals

The learner should complete the learner contract as early as possible, preferably on the first day. After reviewing the learner's goals, you can modify the contract based on your judgment and previous experience. Specific strategies to address the content in the contract can be included. The contract is then reviewed and signed by you and the learner.

Responsibilities

Be as explicit as possible about the entire spectrum of responsibilities. Consider such mundane but important aspects as how to dress, where to park, through what doorway to enter the building, and where to store personal possessions as well as expectations about writing or dictating notes, ordering tests and consultations, and following up with patients. You can save time if these general rules are written down for the learner and reviewed at the beginning of the experience. Remember to save all orientation materials in a file for subsequent learners.

Scheduling

Review the flow of patients through the office and how teaching will occur. For example, beginning students might be asked simply to observe initially, then be allowed to see selected patients on their own, reporting back after a specified time when you and the learner together can see each patient again. Residents may have a schedule of their "own" patients, or other arrangements can be made. For detailed information about scheduling and an example of an effective schedule, *see "Patient Scheduling" on page 25.*

Teaching

You may wish to tell the learner you will "teach on the fly" primarily by asking questions, role modeling, and directing the learner to the literature to answer important content questions. Whatever approach is used, briefly describe what will occur and what the learner must do to make the process work. Models of different case-based–learning techniques are presented later in this book (*see Chapter 5*) and include the information needed to accomplish this task.

Evaluation and Feedback

The learner needs to know about evaluation and feedback, including when and how it will occur and a clear idea of what criteria will be used for evaluation. Use this time to reassure the learner that informal feedback will be offered frequently during the experience, so the results of the final evaluation will not be unexpected. It's often a good idea to set aside time at this point for a mid-rotation feedback appointment. This commits you to providing the feedback and gives the learner specific information on how and when it will take place.

Office Flow

You or your office manager should take a few minutes to provide an orientation to the office. Introduce the learner to all members of the office staff and provide an explanation of their duties and responsibilities. You might consider conducting your introductions in a way that simulates the flow of patients through the office, beginning with the receptionist, medical-record personnel, health aides, nurses, checkout staff, and others.

Examination Rooms

Review the contents of a typical examination room, including the locations of gloves, gowns, stool cards, and examination instruments. If you expect the learner to fill out laboratory or radiology request forms, show the learner where they are located and how to fill them out. Other innovative ways to introduce the learner to an office is to have him or her actually "check in" as a patient. Using this technique, he or she meets the receptionist, fills out medical forms, is ushered into an examination room, is escorted to the laboratory, is given checkout materials, is taken to the checkout window, and is then sent to the laboratory or to the radiology department. There is no educational experience quite like being a patient.

Workspace and Notes

Define, if you can, the learner's workspace, including where they can sit, place their personal belongings, and perform charting. Review your expectations about charting or dictation and telephone and computer use. Show how they can access information, including textbooks, journals, and online materials.

Informing Patients

At the time the learner arrives, post notices for patients about the learner's participation around the reception area and at the front desk (*see "Patient Notice for Students in the Office" and "Patient Notice for Residents in the Office" on pages 118 and 119*). Many practices take photographs of their current learners and place them in the waiting area with the learner's name and title (i.e., student or resident physician). Ask the reception staff to tell patients that you are teaching a student or resident. You might consider creating a short biography of the learners and offering it to patients when they arrive. Patients appreciate this type of personal knowledge about new faces in the office (*see "Biography of a Resident Physician" on page 120*).

❖ Patient Scheduling

Proper patient scheduling for you and the learner can improve office and teaching efficiency. One example of efficient scheduling is the wave schedule (*see "The Wave Schedule" on page 128 and the table on page 26*). This model begins with your usual schedule, but every second or third patient is asked to come to the office one appointment slot earlier, allowing you and the learner to see patients simultaneously. Patients need to be informed that their visit will be a "double visit," because they may have other appointments or meetings scheduled. After the visits are completed, your patient is discharged from the office and then you and the learner examine the second (learner's) patient together during the freed appointment slot. A typical schedule changed to a wave schedule might look like the following table:

WAVE SCHEDULE

Time AM	Original Physician Schedule	Learner Wave Schedule	Physician Wave Schedule
8:00–8:20	Patient A	Patient A	Patient B
8:20–8:40	Patient B	Patient A	Patient A
8:40–9:00	Patient C	Writes note	Patient C
9:00–9:20	Patient D	Patient D	Patient E
9:20–9:40	Patient E	Patient D	Patient D
9:40–10:00	Patient F	Writes note	Patient F
10:00–10:20	Patient G	Patient G	Patient H
10:20–10:40	Patient H	Patient G	Patient G
10:40–11:00	Patient I	Writes note	Patient I
11:00–11:20	Patient J	Patient J	Patient K
11:20–11:40	Patient K	Patient J	Patient J
11:40–Noon	Patient L	Writes note	Patient L

This model allows physicians to see the same number of patients with a learner present, without necessarily extending the day. The wave schedule can be more intense for advanced learners (who can see every other patient) or less intense for novices (who need more time to write notes or read about patients during the day). The training program should provide you with guidelines as to the number of new and return patients the learner is expected to see. Be prepared to modify this when you have ascertained the learner's competency and efficiency. Obviously, this model requires the staff to call and ask selected patients to arrive early for their appointment. This also is an opportunity to explain that a learner is in the office, to inform them of the possibility of an extended visit, and to obtain permission for the learner to see them.

Although this model demonstrates a schedule with appointments every 20 minutes, it is easily adaptable to schedules of any appointment length, provided that the slots are of equal length. In any case, review the schedule with learners at the beginning of each session. Point out who they will see, "prime" them with your expectations for the visit, and "frame" the visit by emphasizing the time limits and your expectations about what parts of the physical examination to perform and how the case is to be presented. (*See "Strategies for Organizing the Office Visit" on page 37 for information about priming, framing, and patient-presentation format.*)

When arranging the learner's schedule, keep in mind his or her level of expertise and previous outpatient experiences. If possible, select patients who match the learner's abilities. Inexperienced learners do best seeing patients with a single, simple problem or patients with classical or typical presentations of common diseases. Also, it is best to select patients who are good historians, are "patient" patients, and who do not have major psychosocial issues. Complex patients can easily overwhelm the novice learner. On the other hand, advanced learners like to be challenged with undifferentiated clinical problems, enabling them to practice in an environment that typifies clinical practice. Patients with multiple, complex medical problems are appropriate for these learners.

Another efficient scheduling model is the "work-in schedule." In this model, the learner is assigned to see a sufficient number of urgent work-in patients to meet the curricular goals of the experience.

Alternatively, you can see the work-in patients and the learner can see some of the regularly scheduled patients if this arrangement better meets with the institution's expectations or with the learner contract.

Keep in mind that there may be other valuable learning experiences for the student, including the following:

- Home visits
- Hospice visits
- Nursing home visits
- Physical therapy visits
- Laboratory/blood drawing experience
- Giving injections (great experience during flu season)
- Patient-education encounters
- Working with the receptionist
- Working with the business manager
- Attending office business meetings
- Triaging patient telephone calls

Although these experiences are not intended to replace the clinical experience in the office, they are often greatly appreciated by the learner as supplemental experiences. It will be more meaningful to the learner if you articulate the rationale for the experience and provide the learner an opportunity to review the experience with you at a later time.

❖ When the Patients Arrive

Have the receptionist inform incoming patients that you are working with a learner today. Some offices prepare an inexpensive brochure or "newsletter" that describes the teaching program and introduces the learner to the patient (*see "Biography of a Resident Physician" on page 120*). Patients appreciate these informational pieces, particularly when they emphasize personal information about the learner. Some institutions will provide these for you and include a photograph of the learner. The receptionist should be prepared to answer any patient questions about the program and the learner in a positive and supportive fashion (*see "When the Patients Arrive Checklist" on page 98*).

Before the learner enters the room, personally inform your patients that you are providing a learning experience in your office for a medical student or resident. Ask the patient's permission before bringing the learner into the examining room or before allowing the learner to see the patient independently. You may wish to ask permission to have the learner give the case findings to you in front of the patient. As discussed later, this technique can save you considerable teaching time and is typically appreciated by the patient (*see "Presenting in the Room" on page 65*).

When introducing the learner, use positive language: "I have a medical student/resident physician working with me today. If it's OK with you, I'd like him/her to talk to you and examine you first. I will come in and see you afterwards." Most patients will react positively, particularly when it is presented by you in an affirmative fashion, and will be comfortable and willing to have the learner in the room. However, never assume this to be the case. Allow each patient to make the final determination.

If you teach frequently, consider informing new patients that you often work with learners. This sets the expectation for the office, even if the individual learners change over time.

Have the office staff inform you about any positive or negative feedback from the patients about the learner. Use this information in your feedback sessions with the learner. Nothing is as powerful as patient feedback to change learner behavior (2).

❖ After the Patients Leave

Whether you are teaching or not, you must document the patient's visit in order to be eligible for reimbursement by Medicare (and other insurance carriers). Lack of proper documentation can lead to charges of Medicare fraud.

Documentation Requirements for a Resident

Current Medicare rules permit a teaching physician (preceptor) to substantiate a bill based on the combination of the resident's and the teaching physician's documentation of a specific service. The teaching physician must clearly convey that he or she saw the patient and participated personally in the patient's care up to the level of the evaluation and management services billed. The teaching physician can confirm that he or she verified the findings in the resident's note and agree with findings as documented by the resident. The teaching physician can also indicate that he or she agrees with the diagnosis and plan as written by the resident. These rules permit a certain amount of time saved by using the resident's documentation as part of your own note. This will somewhat decrease the overall work associated with teaching by allowing you to receive some "service" for your educational endeavors.

Example of a Note by Attending Physician Dr. Smith Who Is Supervising Resident Physician Dr. Fox

I saw Mrs. Jones with Dr. Fox for dizziness associated with standing up quickly. She was recently started on hydrochlorothiazide for hypertension and has no history of blood or fluid loss. She is orthostatic as noted. Her cardiovascular and neurological examinations are normal. I agree that her symptoms are due to hydrochlorothiazide and that a chemistry panel and hematocrit should be done. See Dr. Fox's note as signed by me for more details. [Signed] Dr. Smith.

Documentation Requirements for a Student

The only documentation by medical students that may be used by the teaching physician is the review of systems (ROS) and past, family, and social histories (PFSH). Currently, the teaching physician may not refer to a medical student's documentation of physical examination findings or medical decision making in his or her note. These restrictions obviously will have an effect on office efficiency. However, certain strategies can be used to maximize efficiency in spite of these regulatory requirements. (*See "The Wave Schedule" on page 128 and "Presenting in the Room" and "Collaborative Examinations" on pages 65–67 for other methods to help manage documentation requirements when a student is present.*)

References

1. **Skeff KM.** Enhancing teaching effectiveness and vitality in the ambulatory setting. *J Gen Intern Med.* 1988;3:S26–33.
2. **Cope DW, Linn LS, Leake BD, Barrett PA.** Modification of residents' behavior by preceptor feedback of patient satisfaction. *J Gen Intern Med.* 1986;1:394–8.

4

Teaching Skills and Organizational Techniques for Office-Based Teaching

T his chapter begins with a description of meaningful patient responsibility and an overview of the personal characteristics of outstanding clinical teachers. This is followed by descriptions of useful pre-visit organizational strategies. (*See "Summary of the Learning Experience" on page 99 for an outline of this chapter and Chapters 5 and 6.*)

❖ Meaningful Responsibility

To create a truly effective learning experience, students and residents need meaningful responsibility as providers of health care. The amount of responsibility depends on the learner's level of training and your best judgment. Nevertheless, most learners need the opportunity to see patients independently, collect data, make preliminary decisions, and then report back to you. As the preceptor, you need to balance between having learners "see it all" (with you) and having them working on their own with fewer patients.

Although there is educational merit in having learners watch you interact with patients, if the entire experience is observational, learners grow frustrated and bored. Of course, there is a natural tendency to want learners to be under your direct observation when working in the office. This is stimulated by being concerned about patient satisfaction, wanting to provide care personally, and keeping on schedule. However, as previously noted, patient satisfaction with learners is usually high, and by using the various techniques presented in this text you can personalize your care and minimize delays in your schedule.

❖ Characteristics of Effective Clinical Teachers

Surveys of graduating medical students and residents have been used to describe characteristics that correlate best with overall teaching effectiveness. National teaching experts and direct observation of experienced teachers have confirmed the validity of the survey results (1–6). Excellent ambulatory teachers were described as those physicians who are good at the following actions:

- Communicating expectations
- Stimulating interest enthusiastically
- Interacting skillfully with patients
- Involving the learner in the teaching process
- Role modeling the desired behaviors

Communicating Expectations

As discussed previously, the best time to communicate expectations is during the office orientation. Be as explicit as possible, and organize your orientation by using a checklist (see "When the Learner Arrives Orientation Checklist" on page 96). Assign various staff members responsibilities for different parts of the orientation. Consider asking the learner at the end of the rotation if there was anything else that would have been useful in the orientation. Be willing to modify your orientation procedure based on feedback from your exiting learners.

Stimulating Interest Enthusiastically

Stimulating learner interest is a vital component of establishing a positive learning environment (5). You must allow your natural enthusiasm for patient care to be expressed through your words and actions. Unusual aspects of problems should be shared with the learner, comparisons with past experiences should be made, and invitations for learners to share their reactions should be solicited. Recall that, for the novice learner, all patients present special challenges, and even repetitive patient problems can be stimulating if different aspects of care are highlighted in the discussion. For example, one patient with diabetes can be the springboard for a discussion on natural history, a second could elicit a lesson on prevention, and a third may illustrate compliance issues. Through your actions, the learner will see each patient as being unique and presenting a different opportunity to learn more about medicine.

Interacting Skillfully with Patients

Excellent clinical teachers are knowledgeable and clinically competent, have good rapport with patients, and are perceived as excellent role models (7). You can provide a valuable educational experience to learners by demonstrating a mastery of the traits you acquired through years of experience (8). Occasionally, take advantage of this wealth of talent by having the learner observe you interacting with patients. First, "set the stage" by telling the learner what to look for and why it is important, afterward providing an opportunity for the learner to describe what took place (9). Then observe the learner as he or she takes the opportunity to practice the skill that you have demonstrated and provide feedback. For example, before counseling a patient about smoking cessation, ask the learner to observe you, with the expectation that he or she will counsel the next patient who needs similar information. You will watch the learner's counseling efforts and later provide him or her with a specific evaluation of the performance.

Involving the Learner

Active observation, as described above, is one method of involving the learner. Other methods include having the learner identify his or her own knowledge and skill limitations, then organizing resources to address these deficiencies (2). Learners can be given assignments that address their learning needs and be told to report back with the results of their research.

One useful teaching strategy is the educational prescription (*see "Educational Prescription Form" on page 129*). When a learning issue becomes apparent, you can take a prescription pad and write out the problem or the assignment. For example, "Is a seven-day course of antibiotics superior to a three-day course for an uncomplicated UTI?" or "Read about the treatment of uncomplicated cystitis." The prescription also should denote a time frame for completing the assignment and how it should be completed, e.g., "Provide a five-minute summary of the evidence tomorrow morning" or "Make a five-minute presentation on cystitis by the end of the day."

You can model key attitudes of active inquiry and lifelong learning by demonstrating patient-centered clinical problem solving. This can be done by verbally framing for the learner the clinical question that needs to be answered, such as, "Is finasteride more effective than doxazosin in the treatment of benign prostatic hypertrophy?" Then demonstrate how the question can be answered by using data from the medical literature or other sources of reliable information.

Role Modeling the Desired Behaviors

Role modeling is an integral component of medical education and an important factor in shaping the values, attitudes, behavior, and ethics of learners. In a study of teaching physicians who were identified as excellent role models by internal medicine residents, several characteristics were identified that distinguished them from physicians who were not chosen as role models. Excellent role models were more likely to stress the importance of the doctor-patient relationship, to spend more time on the psychosocial aspects of medicine, and to give more in-depth and specific feedback to learners (10). Excellent role models also were more likely to engage in activities that built relationships with residents (e.g., asking about career plans, family, and outside interests and providing personal information about their lives). Characteristics that were *not* associated with being an excellent role model included age, sex, academic rank, additional education beyond the medical degree, and part-time/full-time status.

This information suggests that all community-based physicians can be excellent role models. The task of being a role model can be made easier by remembering that learners in your office are actually trying on your job and lifestyle "for size." Be an effective advocate for your specialty by demonstrating enthusiasm for what you are doing. Keep in mind that students and residents learn best from watching experts deal with difficult situations. Allow this to happen by inviting the learner in the room when you anticipate such a situation. Afterward, discuss the encounter with the learner to maximize the process. Learners also appreciate the opportunity to see an experienced physician working within a long-term physician-patient relationship. For many, this will be their first experience in this type of setting, and an opportunity to observe your interaction with an established patient will be both educational and motivational.

Comments from students and residents shed further light on good teaching. As expected, effective ambulatory teachers possess a "broad knowledge of medicine," but also good teachers are "good people." As a group, effective teachers enjoy teaching and patient care, demonstrate concern for their patients, are personal and approachable, show respect for others, and are enthusiastic (5).

❖ Strategies for Organizing the Office Visit

Learners in general, and students in particular, often have trouble deciding how to organize the process of collecting and then presenting patient data. Compared with the hospital environment in which time is not a factor, the ambulatory setting presents unique challenges of addressing patient concerns and collecting information in a limited amount of time. The following paragraphs describe tools and tips that can help organize the learner's visit with the patient (*see "Tools To Help the Learner Organize the Patient Visit" on page 124*).

Data Collection and Patient Presentation

One of us (LEP) has created the following organizational scheme for learners at the University of Washington:

What?

> ► Elicit the patient's agenda: "What should we talk about today?"

Why?

> ► Elicit the patient's attribution or understanding of the problem: "What do you think is causing this? What do you think should be done?"

Why?

> ► Identify the most likely hypothesis and supporting data. Be able to answer the question, "What is the supporting evidence?"

What else?

> ► Create a prioritized and weighted differential diagnosis. Again, be able to answer the question, "What is the supporting evidence?"

What now?

> ► Determine the immediate next steps: "What history, parts of the focused examination, and tests need to be done? What are the treatment options? What patient education needs to be done?"

To be used effectively, you should take a few minutes to go over this organizational framework with the learner, possibly during the orientation. To help the learner, this framework is formatted as a series of tables that can be copied and written on to guide the data collection (*see "Tools To Help the Learner Organize the Patient Visit" on page 124*). For learners having trouble making a patient presentation, the "Patient Presentation Format for Learners" in Appendix B also can be used as a guide. The time spent in acclimating the student to the organizational framework and presentation format will be repaid in increased efficiency during the course of the rotation.

Priming

Another organizational strategy that can be used to focus the visit is "priming." Priming involves providing the learner with pertinent patient-specific background information just before seeing the patient and directing the student to perform specific tasks of patient care (11). For example, if a learner is about to see a patient with chest pain, you might *briefly* (for 1–2 minutes) review with the learner the most common causes of chest pain and aspects of the history and physical examination that would be helpful in differentiating between causes. For patients with chronic medical problems, priming might involve reviewing health maintenance or disease screening needs just before the visit. Priming can be used when seeing complex patients with multiple medical problems by having the learner review what might be the most important outcome of the office visit (*see the box below*).

How a Learner May Be Primed for a Visit

▶ "Mrs. Jones is a healthy 28-year-old woman and is here for her yearly examination. At her age, what are the important screening issues to be covered?"

▶ "Mr. Smith is a 50-year-old man with chronic lung disease and is here after a brief hospitalization for pneumonia. What symptoms should we look for today, and what parts of the physical examination should we focus on?"

continued

> ► "Miss Doe is a 60-year-old woman with hypertension treated with hydrochlorothiazide and is here with the complaint of dizziness. In her age group, what are the important considerations in the differential diagnosis? What inquires should we make about her medication?"

A brief discussion before the visit that includes the strategy of priming will avoid the learner performing a complete history and physical examination by focusing on the appropriate examination for the problem at hand in the allotted time.

Priming

> ► Giving the learner critical information to help initiate the visit.

Framing

Another organizational strategy that increases the efficiency of the learner is "framing." Framing is setting parameters for the visit such that the learner will accomplish a focused task. For example, learners can be given specific instructions on what to accomplish during the visit: "I want you to take a history of the patient's chest pain, do a cardiovascular examination, and report back to me in 15 minutes."

You will find that not all learners need to be "primed" or have the visit "framed," but most medical students and beginning residents will benefit from this approach.

Framing

> ► Setting expectations and time limits for what you want the learner to accomplish during his or her time with the patient.

REFERENCES

1. **Wilkerson L, Armstrong E, Lesky L.** Faculty development for ambulatory teaching. *J Gen Intern Med.* 1990;5(Suppl):S44–53.
2. **Skeff KM.** Enhancing teaching effectiveness and vitality in the ambulatory setting. *J Gen Intern Med.* 1988;3(Suppl):S26–33.
3. **Roberts KB.** Educational principles of community-based education. *Pediatrics.* 1996;98:1259–63.
4. **Gjerde CL, Coble RJ.** Resident and faculty perceptions of effective clinical teaching in family practice. *J Fam Prac.* 1982;14:323–7.
5. **Irby DM, Ramsey PG, Gillmore GM, Schaad D.** Characteristics of effective clinical teachers of ambulatory care medicine. *Acad Med.* 1991;66:54–5.
6. **Whitman N, Magill MK.** Is attending a teaching skills workshop worth your time? *Fam Med.* 1998;30:255–6.
7. **Irby DM.** Teaching and learning in ambulatory care settings: a thematic review of the literature. *Acad Med.* 1995;70:898–931.
8. **Loftus TH, McLeod PJ, Snell LS.** Faculty perceptions of effective ambulatory care teaching. *J Gen Intern Med.* 1993;8:575–7.
9. **Epstein RM, Cole DR, Gawinski BA, et al.** How students learn from community-based preceptors. *Arch Fam Med.* 1998;7:149–54.
10. **Wright SM, Kern DE, Kolodner K, et al.** Attributes of excellent attending physician role models. *N Engl J Med.* 1998;339:1986–93.
11. **McGee SR, Irby DM.** Teaching in the outpatient clinic: practical tips. *J Gen Intern Med.* 1997;12(Suppl):S34–40.

5

Case-Based Learning

This chapter first answers the question, "What is case-based learning?" and then presents discussions on the five different forms:
- The Microskills Model
- The "Aunt Minnie" Model
- Modeling Problem Solving
- The One-Minute Observation
- Learner-Centered Precepting

See also Chapter 6 for models on how to make more efficient use of the available time.

❖ What Is Case-Based Learning?

The traditional model of case-based learning is familiar to most physicians. In this model, a learner presents a case to you after independently gathering the patient data. You then must create educational opportunities for the learner that relate to the case and provide care for the patient. These tasks might be accomplished by doing the following:

- Role modeling ("Watch me care for the patient")
- Questioning ("Tell me what you think and why")
- Performing expert consultation ("Ask me what you need to know")
- Mini-lecturing ("I will tell you what I know about this topic")
- Modeling problem solving ("I will think out loud about this case")
- Encouraging self-directed, independent learning ("What do you want to read about?")
- Assigning teacher-directed, independent learning ("I think you should look this up")

❖ The Microskills Model

Several years ago, five rules or microskills of effective teaching were published by Neher and coworkers (1) as a practical model of case-based learning (*see "Summary of the Microskills Model for Precepting" on page 102*). The microskills method combines expert consultation with the technique of questioning to address learner and patient needs efficiently and effectively. This technique has the added benefit of allowing you 1) to assess what the learner does and does not know, 2) to instruct the learner, and 3) to provide feedback more efficiently. The microskills can be used with nearly any level of learner skill. The five rules are:

---

1. Get a commitment
  ▶ "What do you think is going on with this patient?"

2. Probe for supporting evidence
  ▶ "Why do you think that?"

3. Teach general rules
  ▶ "Always do this when you see a similar case"

continued

4. Reinforce what was done right
- ▶ "Here is what you did right, and this is why it is important"

5. Correct mistakes
- ▶ "I will tell you what you did right"
- ▶ "I will tell you what you can do better"
- ▶ "I will tell you how to do it better"

Get a Commitment

The first microskill refers to having the learner commit to some decision or plan of action. The cue to use this microskill is when the learner pauses after presenting a patient, waiting for you to offer an explanation of the findings or a course of action. At this point, instead of solving the problem and inadvertently missing a teaching opportunity, you should ask, "What do you think is going on?" Other appropriate questions might include, "What do you want to do" or "How would you manage this?" Making a commitment encourages the learner to feel more responsible for the patient, forces active participation in learning, and engenders a sense of collaboration with you. It also enhances the processing of the collected information and sheds light on how pieces of information can be synthesized and

Helpful Approaches To Getting a Commitment
- ▶ "What do you think is going on with this patient?"
- ▶ "Why do you think the patient continues to be hypertensive on three medications?"
- ▶ "What do you want to accomplish during this visit?"

These questions are characterized by expecting the learner to offer an explanation, not just answering "yes" or "no"; he or she must elaborate his or her knowledge for you.

Unhelpful Approaches To Getting a Commitment

> ▶ "Sounds like pneumonia, don't you think?"
> ▶ "Can you think of anything else?"
> ▶ "Did you consider CHF the cause of his dyspnea?"

These questions do not demand elaboration of knowledge by the learner; they can be answered "yes" or "no," and the answer is often prompted by the nature of the question.

---

used in decision making. Learners who make mistakes reveal gaps in their knowledge or judgment that can be addressed by you, either with a short explanation or with a follow-up reading assignment.

Probe for Supporting Evidence

Probing for supporting evidence is the next logical step in teaching. The use of this microskill is indicated after the learner makes a commitment, then looks to you for confirmation that the answer was correct. At this point, instead of saying, "You are right" or "You are wrong," ask the learner for the evidence that supports the commitment. Examples of probing questions include, "What were the major findings that led you to that diagnosis?" or "Why did you choose furosemide rather than hydrochlorothiazide?" Probing questions help the learner reflect on the mental steps that were used to make the commitment. It is important to remember that probing for more information is not the same as "grilling" learners, and they should be told that this is a process intended to help them "think out loud" and to facilitate learning. It also gives you a chance to analyze a learner's diagnostic abilities by understanding the mental processes that lead to his or her conclusion. It is important to probe in a way that allows you a window into the learner's knowledge base and problem-solving skills. This is much more useful than having a learner try to guess what you want him or her to say.

Helpful Approaches To Probing for Supporting Evidence

▶ "What about his presentation led you to this diagnosis?"

▶ "How did you decide that Mrs. Smith has pneumonia?"

▶ "What did you find on exam that makes you think this is a surgical abdomen?"

▶ "What were the factors that made you consider esophageal reflux rather than cardiac ischemia?"

These questions are characterized by asking the learner to demonstrate his or her thinking as it pertains to the case at hand. The learner must synthesize collected data and content knowledge to justify the diagnosis.

Unhelpful Approaches To Probing for Supporting Evidence

▶ "What are the possible causes of dyspnea on exertion?"

▶ "I don't think this is PID. Do you have any other ideas?"

▶ "This seems like a clear case of gout to me; how about you?"

▶ "What are the five most common bacterial causes of community-acquired pneumonia?"

These unhelpful questions are characterized by either having the learner create "lists" of diagnoses that may not be pertinent to the patient's problem or are "leading" questions that do not permit thoughtful consideration of the problem.

The skillful use of questions is an important technique used by experienced clinicians to teach and evaluate learners. As with the examination of a patient, you can start with closed-ended questions that allow for a small range of potentially correct answers. As the student's ability increases, the use of open-ended questions allows for broader ranges of potentially correct answers and a deeper probing of knowledge and judgment. Whitman and Schwenk (2) have described five levels of questions useful in teaching and assessment; these are listed in the table on page 48 with illustrative examples. Some of these categories of questions can be incorporated easily into

QUESTIONS USED TO TEACH AND EVALUATE LEARNERS

Type	Examples	Comments
Factual	Who is the patient? Why is the patient here? When did the patient's back pain begin? What is the most common cause of back pain?	Factual questions, for obtaining information and beginning discussions, consist of the five "W"s: who, what, when, where and why. If you find yourself using only factual questions, it probably means you haven't done an adequate job of orienting the student to your presentation needs or the learner hasn't mastered the technique; either way, go back to square one and reassess the process.
Broadening	What are some other causes of back pain?	Broadening questions can be used to assess additional knowledge not elicited by factual questions. This is a useful type of question, but having to use it suggests either that the student wasn't asked to provide a differential diagnosis as part of the presentation or that he or she has not mastered this skill. *Refer the student to the "Patient Presentation Format for Learners" on page 126.* Consider whether you still want the student to present a differential diagnosis for each patient; follow up with the appropriate instructions.
Justifying	What in the patient's history and physical examination supports your diagnosis?	Justifying questions are used to challenge ideas and assess depth of knowledge and understanding. These are excellent probing questions suggested by the microskills teaching model.
Hypothetical	Suppose your patient has a history of prostate cancer. How would that influence your diagnosis?	Hypothetical questions are used to explore new situations and are effective in creating a more diverse patient population for the learner. This type of question can be useful when seeing your tenth patient with a "run of the mill" problem by allowing you to create new learning situations.
Alternative	Suppose we got an MRI scan next week instead of today. What would be the advantages and disadvantages?	Alternative questions can be used to assess decision-making skills by presenting different plans and asking for probable outcomes. Answering this type of question requires a higher order of content mastery and judgment.

the microskills model. The use of other types of questions indicates a poorly performed patient presentation, an ineffective orientation to the task, or both.

Questions coupled with immediate feedback are powerful teaching tools that, with practice, can be mastered by any preceptor. These questions also make excellent evaluation tools. When used sequentially, they allow you to assess the skill level of the learner, i.e., is the learner capable of only reporting the data or can he or she synthesize, justify, and demonstrate good judgment and decision-making skills? (*See the "RIME Evaluation Framework" on page 83 for more information on this evaluation scheme.*)

Teach the General Rule

Whenever possible, attempt to teach the general rule (3,4). When something is taught, it is more memorable and easily transferable to other cases when it is offered as a general rule rather than as a patient-specific plan. Also, be assured that it is not imperative to "teach" something with each patient encounter. If the learner has done well, give positive feedback and skip the formal teaching for a situation that is more appropriate.

Helpful Approaches To Teaching General Rules

- ► "If a young adult has mechanical low-back pain, X-rays are not indicated initially."
- ► "It is helpful to address code status while patients are still healthy so that you can have a meaningful discussion."
- ► "When following up a case of pneumonia, remember that the infiltrates on the chest X-ray might not clear for 4 to 6 weeks. It is best to postpone the follow-up X-ray until after that time."

These questions are characterized by creating "rules of thumb" that can be applied reasonably to similar cases. They are short and to the point. The learner can be challenged to look up the scientific rationale for these rules as an independent learning assignment.

Unhelpful Approaches To Teaching General Rules

- ▶ "Mr. Smith does not need a back X-ray today."
- ▶ "Why don't we discuss code status with Mrs. Jones today?"
- ▶ "Arrange for Mr. Doe to have his repeat chest X-ray at the end of the month."
- ▶ "I always treat pneumonia with two antibiotics because patients seem to do better"
- ▶ "I never give a flu and pneumonia vaccination at the same time. It might make the patient sick"

Unhelpful approaches tend to address a specific problem but do not provide a general approach. They may also represent an unsupported, idiosyncratic approach to patient care. It often takes an insightful physician to recognize that this is taking place and to correct it.

Reinforce What Was Done Right

This is sometimes referred to as "catching the learner doing something well." When the learner does well, reinforce what was done correctly by providing positive feedback. Even learners who are doing well may not recognize which elements of their behavior are helpful and, thus, are the ones that continue. Positive feedback helps promote self-esteem and builds confidence and probably heightens awareness to corrective criticism when it is offered. Positive feedback should not be mistaken for general praise ("You did a good job with that last patient") but should be explicit, reinforcing desired behaviors. Effective positive feedback also includes a probable outcome of the observed behavior and provides a rationale for continuing it. For example, "You were very empathic with that patient, and she responded by providing important information in the history."

Helpful Approaches To Reinforcing What Was Done Right

▶ "You evaluated this in a stepwise fashion and considered the patient's preferences in your suggestions. As a result, she is likely to be compliant with our recommendations."

▶ "You did a good job noting the possible role of medication side effects in the diagnosis. This helped us avoid unnecessary tests."

These statements are characterized by providing specific praise that targets a specific action or behavior and the associated real or potential outcome of that action or behavior.

Unhelpful Approaches To Reinforcing What Was Done Right

▶ "Strong work!"

▶ "You did a great job on that last case."

General praise that does not specify the precise action or behavior that was helpful (or how it was likely to be helpful) characterizes unhelpful feedback. The learner will not know exactly what was good, why it was good, or how to duplicate it.

Correct Mistakes

Learners will make mistakes; when they do, supply corrective feedback. For the feedback to be effective, you must choose an appropriate time and place to present the criticism to the learner. It is useful to begin by having learners review their own performance. Most learners have remarkable insight into their weaknesses and tend to be harder on themselves than their supervisors. Follow up the learner's comments with your own observations. Attempt to frame the observation of the mistake as "not the best" rather than "bad" or "wrong." Then, provide specific guidance on improvement, e.g., by saying "You might be more successful next time this happens if you try..." and by giving them an opportunity to practice.

Helpful Approaches To Correcting Mistakes

► "I agree that Goodpasture's is a possible diagnosis but bacterial sinusitis is much more likely based on disease prevalence and lack of other findings. Next time, consider common conditions first."

► "Your diagnosis is correct, but next time consider the patient's financial circumstances in the choice of medication."

This feedback is characterized by identifying a specific behavior or action that needs correction and what needs to be done to improve the next time.

Unhelpful Approaches To Correcting Mistakes

► "You actually ordered *that?*"

► "I can't believe you know so little for a fourth-year student."

These unhelpful statements are characterized as being vague or judgmental and are not accompanied with advice on how to improve. Avoid these kinds of statements. (*See Chapter 7 for more information on giving feedback.*)

The microskills model of effective teaching is but one of many models of case-based learning that are available (4–6). What makes this model so appealing is that it de-emphasizes the effect of transferring "new knowledge" and showcases everyday patient-management skills that are highly valued by all levels of learners.

What Preceptors Can Accomplish with the Microskills Model

- ▶ Diagnosis of the patient by asking questions
- ▶ Analysis of the learner by getting a commitment and probing for evidence
- ▶ Instruction by providing general rules and feedback

The first two microskills listed on pages 44 and 45 analyze learner knowledge and reasoning by asking for a commitment and by probing for supporting evidence. The last three microskills offer instruction that is individualized to meet the learner's needs (i.e., by teaching general rules, reinforcing what was done right, and correcting mistakes).

❖ The "Aunt Minnie" Model

Traditional case-based teaching, as described previously, involves three basic steps: the learner collects data from the patient, reports the data to you, and through a series of questions and answers creates and prioritizes (with you) a differential diagnosis and plan. Cunningham and coworkers (7) have suggested an alternative model based on pattern recognition, otherwise known as the "Aunt Minnie" model (*see "Summary of the 'Aunt Minnie' Model of Precepting" on page 103*). "Aunt Minnie" is the name used by Sackett and coworkers (8) to describe a process of pattern recognition, i.e., if she dresses and walks like Aunt Minnie, she probably *is* Aunt Minnie, even if you cannot see her face (8). This model is particularly effective when time is short and the case is straightforward. After the learner has collected the data from the patient, he or she is asked to present only the chief complaint and the most likely diagnosis. After this 10- to 30-second encounter, the learner is asked to begin writing the note while you evaluate the patient. When you are finished and the patient is being discharged from the office, the case is briefly discussed with the learner and the medical record is reviewed.

Typically, the learner will report the correct diagnosis and you can confirm this immediately. When the learner is wrong, brief and specific feedback is provided. The whole process of discussion is completed within 1 to 5 minutes. This model seems to be an efficient system to expose learners to common and normal circumstances. It allows you and the learner to see patients more quickly and, therefore, to see more patients. Consequently, the learner develops a greater depth of experience.

Cunningham and coworkers (7) have found that, with persistence, the learner can develop the habit of formulating the diagnosis and mentally summarizing the data that support it. After some initial reluctance to refrain from reporting everything they know about the patient, learners should be able to report only the chief complaint and the most likely diagnosis.

Some educators have expressed concerns that the student or resident will not learn how to do a complete history and physical examination and will be taught to make "snap judgments" rather than to consider carefully all aspects of the case. In defense of "Aunt Minnie," learners in office-based clinical rotations already will have been taught how to perform a complete history and physical examination and will have had the opportunity to practice it in the hospital setting. To this end, the advice of Sackett and coworkers (8) is most illuminating: "The student should be taught to do a complete history and physical examination, and then be taught to never use it." Finally, teaching the skill of pattern recognition can be defended because this is a strategy used by experienced clinicians to evaluate common problems. If this strategy is unsuccessful, you can always return to the beginning, ask the patients more questions, and follow up new clues with an appropriate and focused physical examination. The learner then can see how detailed questioning and a directed examination fit properly into the scheme of caring for patients.

One of the benefits of the "Aunt Minnie" model is the provision of immediate, specific feedback to the learner, e.g., "You are right, the patient has acute otitis media" or "You were mistaken, the patient's tympanic membranes are normal, but the external ear canal is red and swollen; it's probably an external otitis. Go back and look again before the patient leaves the room." Use of short, specific messages as part of the feedback makes learners less likely to feel that they have been subjected to an interrogation or personal criticism.

Factors That Facilitate the "Aunt Minnie" Model's Effectiveness

► The problem should be straightforward.
► The preceptor must see the patient.
► The preceptor must know the diagnosis; if the preceptor is uncertain about the diagnosis, he or she must be willing to admit it.

With practice, the learner will be able to distinguish "Aunt Minnie" cases from those requiring a more detailed presentation and discussion. After examining the patient, the learner can tell you "I have an 'Aunt Minnie'" or "We need to discuss this case." From the learner's clue, you can decide to go with "Aunt Minnie" or select another appropriate case-based–learning technique, such as the microskills model.

❖ Modeling Problem Solving

Another form of case-based learning is modeling problem solving. This technique is particularly helpful when time is a factor or when the case is too sophisticated for the learner (3,4). Modeling problem solving involves nothing more than you "thinking out loud" about the patient. This might include 1) reviewing diagnostic hunches and considering the pros and cons of each or 2) providing a rationale for a diagnostic or treatment decision. You can do this with the learner before entering the examination room or in front of the patient. Many patients report that they appreciate hearing their case discussed with learners, because it adds to their own understanding (*see "Presenting in the Room" on page 65*).

This is a passive form of learning, but it can be a valuable way to demonstrate how an expert clinician synthesizes data, prioritizes hunches, and plans the diagnostic and treatment components of care. In a sense, it is what you are asking the learner to do when using the microskills. When you model problem solving, you make a vocal commitment, provide supporting data from the history and physical examination, and might even have time to teach a general rule.

❖ The One-Minute Observation

This is a powerful, case-based, educational strategy proposed by Ferenchick and coworkers (9). It describes how to conduct a brief observation of a learner performing a specific clinical skill, such as collecting part of a history or performing part of the physical examination. Over time, and through the use of several "one-minute observations," much of the learner's history taking and physical examining can be observed (*see "Summary of the One-Minute Observation" on page 104*). This process allows you to observe, first hand, the learner's level of performance without the commitment of large blocks of time. The steps involved in successfully using this strategy are:

- Explaining the purpose of the observation to the learner
- Explaining how the observation will occur
- Informing the patient of your plan and purpose
- Observing for a brief period of time without interrupting
- Leaving the room and having the learner join you when finished with the patient
- Providing immediate feedback
- Using the information gained to plan your teaching

The advantage of this strategy is the opportunity it affords you to observe the clinical skills of the learner. Feedback is then guided by first-hand data, rather than by assumption of skill level based on the patient presentation. The process is focused, time efficient, and reassuring to the patient. Furthermore, learners at all levels appreciate the opportunity to receive feedback, and this particular technique is well received by them. Some preceptors have created a checklist for the major parts of the history or physical examination they wish to observe first hand. Over time, each item on the list is observed and checked off (or a notation is made next to the item so that it can be referred to when providing feedback at a later time).

Closely related to the one-minute observation is the "mini-goals" model used by one of us (DED) and Doug Paauw at the University of Washington. In this model, you ask the learner to focus on a specific learning task for the day or week. For example, "Today let's work on history-taking skills. I'll watch you do just the history on one or two patients today and then give you feedback." You then watch the learner perform that task and provide specific instructive comments. At subsequent teaching sessions, the two of you may agree to work on different skills, such as the physical examination, patient education, or the visit "wrap-up." This technique tends to focus the precepting, to increase specific feedback, and to allow the learner to master a specific task or skill.

❖ Learner-Centered Precepting

Learner-centered precepting relies on the learner initiating interactions with you to achieve the following goals:
- Using active involvement to enhance the learning experience
- Teaching patient-centered care more effectively by modeling the process through the teaching encounter
- Addressing learner needs more accurately
- Demonstrating techniques to improve doctor-patient communication through modeling of preceptor-learner communication and negotiation

The use of learner-centered precepting uses the same principles as those used in the microskills model but makes the process more explicit. This technique allows the learner to identify what he or she needs to learn and helps you tailor instruction to meet these needs (*see "Summary of Learner-Centered Precepting" on page 105*).

By performing learner-centered precepting, you are modeling the technique that physicians use in patient-centered care, which begins with eliciting the patient's agenda and attribution of the problem. Similarly, learner-centered precepting begins with the learner's statement of agenda and attribution of the learning needs associated with the patient's care. This will help you to asses the learner's understanding and to focus the teaching. This process may help address the documented discordance between what is being taught and what the learner wants to know (10).

This model of case-based learning begins with a patient presentation by the learner that consists of the three parts discussed in the box below.

Identification

▶ The learner first presents the patient-identifying data, visit status (new or return), and the chief complaint. This is also the point at which the learner makes an assessment of his or her general teaching need for this specific patient encounter.

Information

▶ This part addresses the clinical information you need to teach and care for the patient, including a concise history, the results of the physical examination's pertinent parts, the most likely diagnosis, and an initial plan.

Issues

▶ The last part consists of learner-formulated questions about knowledge, skills, or logistical information needed by the learner to care for the patient.

By using this technique, the learner is taught to identify their questions about the case at the beginning of the case presentation. For example, the learner might report (either inside or outside of the examination room), "I'm seeing Mrs. Smith who has type 1 diabetes, and my question is 'Should she have intensive insulin therapy using an insulin pump?'" A question this sophisticated indicates a higher level of learner knowledge than a question such as "Is a blood sugar of 300 OK?" and helps determine your teaching approach as you listen to the remainder of the presentation. The learner who asks the first question obviously has different teaching needs and capabilities compared with the learner who asks the second question. Although this technique is usually helpful, it can be misleading because learners sometimes use medical jargon without completely understanding its application. This technique also will give you a starting point for discussion if you disagree with the learner's perception of the case. For example, you might say, "I understand you want to discuss the use of an insulin pump, but first we need to figure out why the sugars are so high."

To be effective, the learner needs to be instructed on how to frame their questions at the beginning of the presentation and be given positive feedback when done correctly. You must remember to respond to the question during the discussion of the case or to demonstrate or guide the learner toward finding the answer on his or her own.

Learner-centered precepting requires that you orient the learner to your expectations and that you remain consistent. "Up-front" identification of the learning issue by the learner is a more active approach and is more work; thus, unless given a reminder, the learner may not do it consistently. However, learners who use this technique report that it assists them in organizing their thoughts and decreases the mismatch between what they need to know and what the preceptor is teaching.

❖ Pitfalls of Case-Based Learning

There are certain pitfalls inherent in case-based teaching that reduce its effectiveness. The most commonly encountered problems include the following:

- Taking over the case
- Not allowing sufficient "wait time"
- Giving inappropriate lectures
- Asking questions with "preprogrammed answers"
- Pushing the learner past his or her ability

Taking Over the Case

Taking over the case is one of the most common and educationally destructive pitfalls of case-based learning. Typically, this is most likely to occur when a learner gives an incorrect answer to one of the microskills questions (e.g., "What do you think is going on?"). Rather than probing further to find what the learner knows or where the learner has gone astray in the diagnostic reasoning process, the preceptor takes control. The learner is told the diagnosis, what investigations to order, medications to prescribe, and any follow-up plans to pursue. At best, the learner becomes a scribe, taking notes to follow up on the preceptor's suggestions and, at worst, becomes a passive bystander with no role in the case management and no opportunity to learn.

Not Allowing Sufficient "Wait Time"

Closely related to taking over the case is not allowing sufficient "wait time" when asking the learner a question. Physicians have a tendency, whether dealing with patients or learners, to interrupt and ask another question or provide the answer to the first question when an answer is not immediately forthcoming. Having discovered that impatience discourages any real attempt on the part of the learner to answer the question, effective teachers allow the learner more time to consider the question and to formulate a response. When preceptors answer their own questions, learners are quick to recognize that they are not really expected to answer the question and do not put forth the effort. Alternatively, learners working with patient preceptors who wait for an answer learn not only that an answer is expected—even if it is wrong—but also that it is an essential and expected component of the learning process.

Giving Inappropriate Lectures

Another common problem with case-based learning is giving inappropriate lectures. It is inefficient and ineffective to vocalize large amounts of information when it can be researched more easily and with greater educational impact at a later time. As presented in the microskills model, teaching can be given in small "bites" of information. These small "bites" include teaching the general rule and relating it to the immediate situation. For example, "For most young, healthy individuals with back pain, ordering a back X-ray is not cost effective; therefore, we will not order it for Mr. Smith. He fits the profile of patients who do not benefit from an X-ray." The learner can be directed to the primary information sources that support this general rule, and any follow-up reading can be done at a later time. The primary data supporting the general rule should not be presented by you in the form of a mini-lecture.

Asking Questions with "Preprogrammed Answers"

As suggested in the microskills section, preceptors must learn not to ask questions with "preprogrammed answers" that immediately suggest the correct answer, thereby preventing any thinking on part of the learner. An example of a question with a "preprogrammed answer" is "What do you think is going on? Could it be gastritis?" The answer is obvious; it requires no problem solving or data synthesis on part of the learner, and it deprives you of the ability to assess the learner's knowledge and problem-solving skills.

Pushing the Learner Past His or Her Ability

Another common problem with case-based learning is pushing the learner past his or her ability. This usually takes the form of discussing the ramifications of a case beyond his or her comprehension of what is being said or asked. An example would be asking a learner about the advantages of using an angiotensin-converting–enzyme inhibitor in a hypertensive patient with diabetes when he or she has not yet learned about diabetic nephropathy. The key to knowing you have pushed beyond the learner's ability is observing the reaction to your question. Lack of response, lack of follow-up questions, or a neutral facial expression typically signal incomprehension. At this point, the best strategy is assessing what the learner *does* know by using probing questions. Do not to ask questions that can be answered with a simple "yes" or "no" (e.g., "Do you know what diabetic nephropathy is?") but ones that require the learner to explain and synthesize information (e.g., "What do you recall about the effects diabetes has on the kidney?").

The following illustrates a series of probing questions that can help assess the learner's grasp of content:

- "What is the relationship between long-standing hyperglycemia and kidney function?
- "What is the proposed mechanism?"
- "How can it be prevented?"

❖ Concluding the Visit

Regardless of the teaching model used, take time at the end of the visit to review with the learner his or her follow-up responsibilities. These might include the following tasks:

- Arranging for a follow-up appointment, consultation, imaging study, or laboratory work
- Performing vaccinations and other health-maintenance and screening procedures

- Educating patients
- Writing or dictating a chart note
- Updating the "Problem List," "Medication List," and "Health Maintenance/Screening Form"
- Finding data absent from the chart (e.g., laboratory work, consultation, previous note)
- Making "to do" notes (e.g., follow-up telephone call with patient)
- Taking on an independent learning assignment, if appropriate

You might make a note of the patients seen by the learner. This will remind you to follow up with the learner on such things as laboratory results, consultations, and results of therapeutic interventions. Such notes could be kept on a copy of the daily schedule and saved as a patient log for you and the learner. Viewed over time, this information is also useful in determining the adequacy of the learner's experience in terms of numbers of patients seen and their medical and social diversity. It also will help remind you of things the learner has done well and other incidents when you are completing the end-of-rotation evaluation.

REFERENCES

1. **Neher JO, Gordon KC, Meyer B, Stevens N.** A five-step "microskills" model of clinical teaching. *J Am Board Fam Prac.* 1992;5:419–24.
2. **Whitman NA, Schwenk TL.** *Preceptors as Teachers.* Salt Lake City, UT: University of Utah School of Medicine; 1984.
3. **Loftus TH, McLeod PJ, Snell LS.** Faculty perceptions of effective ambulatory care teaching. *J Gen Intern Med.* 1993;8:575–7.
4. **McGee SR, Irby DM.** Teaching in the outpatient clinic: practical tips. *J Gen Intern Med.* 1997;12(Suppl):S34–40.
5. **Wilkerson L, Armstrong E, Lesky L.** Faculty development for ambulatory teaching. *J Gen Intern Med.* 1990;5(Suppl):S44–53.
6. **Skeff KM.** Enhancing teaching effectiveness and vitality in the ambulatory setting. *J Gen Intern Med.* 1988;3(Suppl):S26–33.

7. **Cunningham AS, Blatt SD, Fuller PG, Weinberger HL.** The art of precepting: Socrates or Aunt Minnie? *Arch Pediatr Adolesc Med.* 1999;153:114–6.
8. **Sackett DL, Haynes RB, Tugwell P.** *Clinical Epidemiology: A Basic Science for Clinical Medicine,* 1st ed. Boston: Little, Brown; 1985.
9. **Ferenchick G, Simpson D, Blackman J, et al.** Strategies for efficient and effective teaching in the ambulatory care setting. *Acad Med.* 1997;72:277–80.
10. **Laidley TL, Braddock CH, Fihn SD.** Did I answer your question? Attending physicians' recognition of residents' perceived learning needs in ambulatory settings. *J Gen Intern Med.* 2000;15:46–50.

6

Ways To Be More Efficient When Teaching

This chapter presents five strategies that can be used to become more efficient or to make up lost time in the office, namely:

- Presenting in the Room
- Collaborative Examinations
- Active Observation
- Service-Based Education
- Self-Directed (Independent) Learning

❖ Presenting in the Room

Traditionally, learners report their findings to the teacher outside of the examination room. If you use this model, the next step involves returning to the room to verify the history and physical examination and to plan the care for the patient. A time-saving step would be to have the learner present the patient's case in the examining room in front of the patient. Due to concerns of patient acceptance, preceptors have not adopted this technique universally. However, recent studies show that patients actually approve of this strategy.

Patients report that, with "bedside" presentations (in this case, inside the examination room), doctors spent more time with them and offered better explanations of their problems. Such presentations did not provoke worry, and patients were satisfied with the overall process (1,2). It is important, however, that the learner alert you of any potentially sensitive issues or serious diagnoses being considered before making the presentation. As always, these issues must be handled with care and sensitivity. The learners must be told this and become aware of the power of their words.

Despite high patient acceptance and the obvious time-saving benefits for you, not all learners are comfortable presenting in the room (2), and they may have to be convinced of its value. Some of the benefits of presenting in the room include the following:

- It saves time
- Patients perceive in-the-room presentations as being more confidential than "hallway talk"
- Patients are not waiting alone for the doctors
- Patients prefer to hear what is being said about them
- Learners tend to make more concise presentations
- Patients can verify information
- Patients can correct misinformation
- It increases the preceptor's "face-to-face" time with the patient
- The preceptor can immediately collect additional information that flows naturally from the learner's presentation
- Patients feel they are part of the process
- It helps maintain compliance with the Health Care Financing Administration (HCFA) regulations on billing for services that need to be performed personally by the physician

Despite the enthusiasm of most patients and preceptors about in-the-room presentations, not all discussion between the preceptor and learner should be in front of the patient. Analyzing the learner's thought processes or discussing the differential diagnosis are more suited for private conversations, particularly if they are likely to include entities that are emotionally charged. Discussions of pathophysiology or debates about the literature are best reserved for out-of-room presentations.

Notwithstanding reassurances about the educational value and efficiency of bedside presentations, some learners will be resistant. In these cases, we do not suggest that you abandon in-the-room presentation, because it presents a good opportunity to role model clinical skills and to involve patients in the decision-making process. This may be your best opportunity to demonstrate empathy, compassion, and concern and to validate the usefulness of a skillfully taken history and a focused examination. If this strategy works for you, simply make it happen.

❖ Collaborative Examinations

Collaborative examinations involve the learner and preceptor seeing the patient simultaneously. This technique is most time efficient when working with students. The student takes the lead in taking the history, with you observing. The student is given a defined amount of time to accomplish the task. After the student has completed the history, you can ask any additional questions, with the student observing. Then, the student can be assigned certain parts of the examination to be performed under your direct observation, followed by you repeating parts of the examination to verify essential findings. This technique is useful when attempting to gauge a new learner's level of expertise. It also can be used when formally evaluating a learner or simply to save time. Finally, collaborative examinations offer an excellent opportunity to role model clinical skills and, like presenting in the room, help maintain compliance with the HCFA regulations on billing for services that need to be performed personally by the physician.

❖ Active Observation

Active observation is a useful technique for both students and residents when time is a factor or when the complexity of the problem is too sophisticated for the learner (*see "Summary of Active Observation" on page 106*). In active observation, the learner is asked to observe you performing a clinical skill. The skill may be communication, interviewing, physical examination, or some other procedure.

Active Observation Is Not Shadowing

Care must be taken not to transform this exercise into mere "shadowing," which makes the learner a passive participant. Observation can become an active learning process by "priming" the learner, i.e., describing what will happen, why it needs to happen, and what to look for. Follow up the session with an opportunity for the learner to describe what happened and to practice what was just learned. For active observation to be effective, the following must occur:

- The learner needs to be informed about the rationale for the observation.

   Example: "This patient is very hostile, and I want you to watch how I manage this situation."

- The learner should be told what to observe.

   Example: "Notice how I diffuse his anger by labeling and validating his emotions."

- The learner should be provided with an opportunity to review what was learned after the session.

   Example: "Tell me what you saw when I interviewed the patient."

The learner should be observed practicing what was taught and should be provided feedback on his or her performance. In one study of students, 70% responded that active observation was the most important learning event in their ambulatory medicine rotation (3).

Summary of the Critical Elements in Active Observation

▶ Describing the rationale for the observation ("You should watch me do this because...")

▶ Declaring what the learner should observe ("Watch how I ...")

▶ Reviewing what was observed ("What did you see happen in that session?")

▶ Allowing the learner an opportunity to practice ("When you see the next patient, I want you to...")

❖ Service-Based Education

Service-based education can be an effective teaching strategy for students. It consists of identifying tasks that typically are performed by a member of the office staff (or occasionally by you) and training the student to perform those tasks. This is not to suggest that service-based education can replace the clinical encounter as the main focus of office-based teaching, rather it is meant to supplement the clinical encounter. The advantages to the learner are 1) the opportunity to gain knowledge about and perform tasks that are often critical to the efficient operation of an office and 2) to develop a sense of being a contributing member of the office team. The benefits to the office can be significant, e.g., a student may be able to "free up" a member of the office staff for a period to time to accomplish other tasks. Some of the tasks that students can perform while in the office setting include the following:

- Counseling and education of patients
- Helping to register patients
- Retrieving laboratory or radiology results
- Making follow-up telephone calls
- Triaging patient calls
- Filling out laboratory, radiology, and consultation request forms

- Administering vaccinations
- Conducting patients to the examination room, documenting the reason for the visit, recording vital signs
- Performing electrocardiography
- Sterilizing equipment
- Performing simple office laboratory tests
- Filing and retrieving charts
- Answering clinical questions by using databases (e.g., MEDLINE)

The main idea behind service-based education is not to reduce your office overhead by taking advantage of the student's services but rather to introduce the student to the tasks, talents, and time necessary to run an office. Some of the tasks (e.g., filing and retrieving charts) may require only an hour or two to accomplish, whereas others (e.g., triaging patient telephone calls) may require several hours of dedicated time to capture the complexity and importance of the task. In any event, service-based education is a supplement to, not a replacement of, clinical encounters and patient-based learning.

❖ Self-Directed (Independent) Learning

When there is a lull in the office (e.g., lunch time, end of the day), ask the learner a few questions that stimulate reflection and promote self-directed learning (4-6) (*see "Summary of Self-Directed [Independent] Learning" on page 107*). Such questions might include the following:

- "Based on the patients you saw today, what are your questions?"
- "What did you learn today?"
- "What was the most important thing that happened today?"
- "What is the one thing you would like to learn more about?"
- "What troubled you today?"
- "What might you improve on?"

Considering role modeling this behavior by indicating what *you* learned today, what questions were generated for you, and how you intend to answer them. By role modeling the behavior, you demonstrate the importance of this approach to continuing education. You also can use this time to ask the learner to participate in some self-directed learning.

The two essential steps in self-directed learning are the identification of the limits of one's knowledge and skills and the ability to organize resources to learn more (7). Self-directed study engages the learner in critical thinking and hands-on experiences that promote application of book knowledge to "real world" experiences. Self-directed learning also can promote the study of diseases and conditions that the learner is unlikely to see at the office due to case mix and prevalence.

To maximize effectiveness, self-directed learning should be linked to a recently observed patient problem. The opportunity to store knowledge in the context from which it will be retrieved (i.e., case-based learning) aids the learning process (8). Additionally, reading around recently encountered cases is more motivating than asking learners to tackle the textbook chapter by chapter.

Self-directed learning is a reasonable learning goal for either the student or resident. If learning resources are available in the office, learners can be asked to pursue questions that remain unanswered after a patient visit, with the understanding that the information will be conveyed back to you at a later but specifically defined time. For example, a convenient review time might be at the end of the day after all the patients have been seen. Also, asking the learner to pursue unanswered questions through independent reading is a technique that can be used to help you "catch up" when you are behind in your schedule. While the learner is reading, you can see one or two patients independently.

The following box summarizes the main components of self-directed learning; this can be used as a checklist when making assignments for learners in the office:

Identify the Learner Need

▶ After hearing the case presentation (or at the end of the session), either have the student identify his or her learning question or prompt the student by asking "What bothers you most about this case?"

Make an Assignment

▶ The learner is asked to formulate the learning question, research the question, and report back to you.

Identify resources

▶ Potential resources include textbooks, journal articles, consultants, and MEDLINE and other electronic databases.

"Close the loop"

▶ Have the learner report back to you on what was found, either vocally, in a written outline, or incorporated in a patient write-up or assessment.

The educational prescription is a tool that can help both you and the learner formalize the process of self-directed learning (*see "Educational Prescription Form" on page 129*).

REFERENCES

1. **Lehmann LS, Brancati FL, Chen MC, et al.** The effect of bedside case presentations on patient's perceptions of their medical care. *N Engl J Med.* 1997;336:1150–5.
2. **Wang-Cheng RM, Barnas GP, Sigmann P, et al.** Bedside case presentations: why patients like them but learners don't. *J Gen Intern Med.* 1989;4:284–7.
3. **Epstein RM, Cole DR, Gawinski BA, et al.** How students learn from community-based preceptors. *Arch Fam Med.* 1998;7:149–54.
4. **Arseneau R.** Exit rounds: a reflection exercise. *Acad Med.* 1995;70:684–87.

5. **DaRosa DA, Dunningham GL, Stearns J, et al.** Ambulatory teaching "lite": less clinic time, more educationally fulfilling. *Acad Med.* 1997;72:358–61.

6. **Smith CS, Irby DM.** The roles of experience and reflection in ambulatory care education. *Acad Med.* 1997;72:32–5.

7. **Skeff KM.** Enhancing teaching effectiveness and vitality in the ambulatory setting. *J Gen Intern Med.* 1988;3(Suppl):S26–33.

8. **Bordage G.** Elaborated knowledge: a key to successful diagnostic thinking. *Acad Med.* 1994;70:883–5.

7

Learner Feedback and Evaluation

This chapter addresses the relationship between assessment, feedback, and evaluation. It presents useful tips on how to provide effective feedback and systematically evaluate a learner, describes a useful evaluation model, and summarizes how to avoid evaluation errors.

❖ What Are Some Effective Methods of Learner Feedback?

Feedback is information provided to learners about their current clinical performance that is intended to guide their future clinical performance (1–3) (*see "Summary of Feedback" on page 108*). Feedback is based on an assessment of the learner's knowledge, attitude, and skills observed during the office rotation. Feedback can be positive or negative, describing appropriate or inappropriate actions or behaviors. Feedback should be constructive, consisting of a combination of positive and negative comments with a description of how to improve next time. Learners desire constructive feedback. The complaint heard most frequently from learners is that no one tells them how they are doing. What learners fear most is destructive feedback, statements that are made in a way that punishes, belittles, or embarrasses them. Unfortunately, this is an experience that is all too common.

Feedback is important because it tells the learner what he or she is doing right and wrong and points out what needs to be accomplished to get to the next level of proficiency. Studies have shown that intensive feedback provided to residents significantly improves their patient-satisfaction scores compared with residents who did not receive feedback (4). Ideally, feedback should be given every time you interact with a learner, but realistically this is seldom possible. At a minimum, you should offer feedback at regular intervals during the learning experience. Constructive feedback has several identifiable qualities that are described in the table on page 77.

Studies of effective feedback techniques have verified the usefulness of the feedback "sandwich" (5), which has three components delivered in the following order:

- What was done right
- What was done wrong
- What to do next time

When you begin with a positive comment, the learner is more receptive to subsequent messages in the "meat" of the feedback sandwich, which is composed of corrective feedback—things the learner did not do well and needs to improve. When describing the observed behavior, be as specific as possible. Finally, end the feedback with detailed instructions for improvement and remember to follow up with positive feedback and praise if the learner is able to meet this objective. The box on page 78 contains examples of short, relevant feedback sandwiches.

Feedback is more effective with a little advanced planning. Inform the learner at the beginning of the rotation that feedback will be provided throughout the experience. Select an appropriate time and place and provide it privately as soon as possible after the learning event. Select only one or two important items to discuss, and keep the discussion to approximately five minutes or less. Serve the "feedback sandwich," be sure that the learner understands what has been said, and arrange for a follow-up.

CONSTRUCTIVE FEEDBACK

Quality	Comment	Good Example	Poor Example
Descriptive, not evaluative	Describes the behavior you observe without attributing value to it	"You did not make eye contact with the last patient during the interview"	"You are not interested in patient care" "Your personality is not suitable for a physician"
Specific, not general	Identifies the precise behavior you wish to highlight, avoiding generalities	"You were able to convey empathy and understanding during the interview"	"You did a good job" "You could have done better"
Focused on issues the learner can control	Provides tips on how to improve	"When taking the history, speak slower and check for understanding"	"My patients cannot understand you because of your accent"
Well timed	Makes feedback an expectation, not an exception	When it is provided regularly throughout the learning experience and as close as possible to the event that brought about the feedback	When it is provided only at the end of the rotation
Limited in amount	Make the message memorable	When it focuses on a single, important message	When the learner is overwhelmed with information
Addresses learner goals	Refers back to the learner contract (see Chapter 3 and "Learner Contract" on page 116) or other information gathered during the orientation	When it addresses goals that were identified by the learner at the beginning of the office experience	When the learner's goals are ignored

Relevant Feedback "Sandwiches"

▶ "I like the way you examined the heart. You were method-
ical, going through each step of inspection, palpation, per-
cussion, and auscultation. However, I noticed that you
used only the diaphragm of the stethoscope and not the
bell. The bell is important when listening for low-pitched
sounds. On subsequent patients, I want you to listen with
the bell at each major area."

▶ "Patients seem to like you. Yet, some patients seem to be
frustrated when you don't give them enough time to
answer your questions. Be patient. Wait several seconds,
check to see if they have anything they would like to
add, and then move on."

❖ What Are Some Effective Methods of Learner Evaluation?

An evaluation assigns a value to the learner's performance (*see
"Summary of Evaluation" on page 110*) that is not necessarily an
alphabetical or numerical grade; it can be descriptive, either oral or
written. The value placed on the learner's performance typically is
based on the goals established for the learning experience. The learner performance is judged against the learning goals, and comparisons
are made to these expectations.

In a real sense, evaluation occurs throughout the educational
experience. It is in the assessment (observing) and evaluation (assigning value) process that you generate and provide feedback to the
learner. Under ideal circumstances, assessing, evaluating, and giving
feedback all take place after each learner-patient encounter but can
be provided more realistically as time permits.

In contrast to recognizing the evaluation as part of an ongoing
process of assessment, evaluation, and feedback, most preceptors
equate evaluation with assigning a grade at the end of the rotation. In
keeping with this concept, this section addresses aspects of the final
(or summative) end-of-rotation evaluation.

Typically, medical schools and residency programs collect summative evaluations from preceptors and faculty to meet the following educational needs:

- Identifying learner strengths and weaknesses
- Determining learner competence
- Making decisions about retention and promotion
- Providing information to outside institutions
- Maintaining accreditation of the institution
- Providing legal documentation

Most training programs provide a set of learning goals and objectives that should be reviewed with the learner at the beginning of the office experience. Associated with these learning goals and objectives are the desired knowledge, attitudinal, and skill competencies listed on the institution's evaluation form. The rating scale on the evaluation form measures the degree to which the learner mastered the learning goals and objectives (i.e., the value of the learner's performance). It is a good idea to share the evaluation form with the learner at the beginning of the experience, giving him or her advanced notice of what will be evaluated.

Typically, you will be asked to rate each competency using a predefined scale that can be accompanied by explanatory or illustrative comments. To fill out the form accurately, you must have a sound and efficient method of collecting performance data; use one or more of the following assessment methods:

- Direct observation of learner performance
- Written records (e.g., progress notes, histories, physical-examination findings)
- Patient presentations by the learner
- Responses to probing, hypothetical, and alternative types of questions
- "Homework" assignments
- Interactions with office staff
- Patient comments or measures of satisfaction
- Learner self-evaluation

The most reliable method of collecting performance data is direct observation, i.e., watching the learner take a history, perform an examination, and counsel a patient. Rather than observing a learner-patient interaction from beginning to end, it may be more efficient to observe the learner performing parts of the examination on different patients over time (*see "The One-Minute Observation" on page 56 and "Summary of the One-Minute Observation" on page 104*). For example, over several days, you may observe the learner taking a focused history on one patient, performing a cardiovascular examination on a second patient, and counseling a third.

The learner's progress notes can be reviewed for clarity, accuracy, and understanding of the assessment and plan. Also, charting can be assessed for organization, adherence to the accepted format, completeness, and timeliness.

Following the presentation of the patient by the learner, you can assess the learner's ability to synthesize and present data in a concise and helpful manner. The learner's knowledge and judgment can be evaluated by using the teaching microskills (*see Chapter 5*). The process of having the student make a commitment, followed by probing for supporting information, is an efficient evaluation and teaching technique. By using hypothetical and alternative questioning techniques (*see the box on page 81*), you can assess depth of knowledge.

Observing how the learner interacts with other members of the office staff and soliciting their comments can provide other sources of important evaluation data. Patients are another good source of primary data, and their comments can be collected formally (by asking them to fill out a written survey; *see "Patient Satisfaction Form" on page 130*) or informally (by asking them some casual questions) (6,7). Patient feedback is a powerful motivating factor for modifying learner behavior (4).

Use of a Hypothetical Question

► "I agree that three days of sulfamethoxazole-trimetho-prim is an appropriate choice for this young woman with cystitis. How would you modify your treatment if she were diabetic with a fever and flank pain?"

Use of an Alternative Question

► "What might be the expected outcome if we treated her cystitis with ampicillin rather than sulfamethoxazole-trimethoprim?"

Learners should be expected to follow up on reading and other assignments, and their compliance and thoroughness can be reflected in the evaluation. Finally, learners can perform a self-assessment by filling out a copy of the institution's evaluation form. This self-assessment exercise provides information on the learner's insight and is an excellent opportunity to begin a discussion with the learner about his or her performance.

If you have concerns about a learner's knowledge base, skills, or professionalism, *contact the program early in the process!* Program and clerkship directors can tell you if this is a new or recurring problem, help you resolve the issue, or at least help you and the learner deal with the possibility of a bad evaluation.

❖ What Are the Common Types of Evaluation Errors?

Physicians who rate learners are prone to make one or more rating errors. Some of the errors are understandable given the natural reluctance to submit a poor evaluation that may adversely affect promotion or retention in the training program. Other errors reflect a poor understanding of the evaluation system and its role in identifying sub-optimal performance at a time when remediation is most effective. Common rating errors include:

- The "halo/horn" effect
- Restriction of range
- Rating nonperformance attributes

The "Halo/Horn" Effect

The "halo/horn" effect describes an evaluation bias that is based primarily on the learner's past ratings, not on an objective evaluation of current performance. For example, you have heard through the grapevine that the learner has demonstrated excellent performance in previous rotations and this information influences you to submit an excellent evaluation that may not accurately reflect the actual performance in your office. For example, "Dr. Smith said the student was terrific; maybe my expectations for the student are just too high" or, conversely, "The other preceptors say that he is a terrible resident; maybe I should give him a lower grade."

Not uncommonly, susceptibility to the halo/horn effect is the result of preceptor inexperience or a lack of confidence. It is always best to trust your instincts and make your evaluation based on your observations, not your expectations. Document your decisions whenever possible with specific examples of behaviors that support them. This will allow you to justify the evaluation not only to others but also to yourself.

Restriction of Range

Restriction of range refers to the tendency to circle the same numerical rating for all competencies, thus not making full use of the provided evaluation range. For example, on a five-point scale representing performance attributes from "unsatisfactory" to "superior," the preceptor circles the same score for all the characteristics being evaluated. Although efficient for the preceptor, this rating strategy increases the chances of submitting an inaccurate evaluation. To avoid this error, the preceptor needs to take the time to consider each characteristic individually and rate it independently.

Rating Nonperformance Attributes

Taking into consideration nonperformance attributes when evaluating a competency is another source of error. A bright student who has mastered the cognitive competencies but who is frequently lazy needs to have this attribute reflected in the attitudinal competency section, not the cognitive section of the evaluation. Precisely identifying the categories of poor performance has important implications for learner remediation. Obviously, a remediation program focused on enhancing content knowledge would be wasted on a learner whose attitude needs improvement.

Note: The halo/horn effect and restriction of range are unlikely errors when using a descriptive and developmental evaluation model like the RIME evaluation framework (*see section below*). However, for all its shortcomings, you probably will be given an evaluation form asking you to rate various knowledge, attitude, and skill attributes with a numerical scale. Nevertheless, the RIME model is so simple and intuitive that you can use it to help guide your personal evaluation of the learner. Then, later, you can translate the results of your RIME evaluation to whatever format the sponsoring institution requires.

❖ The RIME Evaluation Framework

A useful framework to guide performance expectations and feedback for office-based learning has been suggested by Pangaro (8) (*see "Summary of the RIME Evaluation Framework" on page 111*). His model integrates learner achievement, provides a framework for putting learner problems in perspective, and is easy to articulate and apply. RIME is a mnemonic for the progressively complex and sophisticated clinical skills shown in the box on page 84.

Reporter

> ► One who can collect and report data.

Interpreter

> ► One who can interpret history clues, physical-examination findings, and laboratory results; can create a problem list; and can prioritize a differential diagnosis

Manager

> ► One who can select the most appropriate diagnostic and treatment options to meet the patient's needs

Educator

> ► One who can identify and address knowledge gaps

The RIME model differs from other evaluation models in that it is "synthetic." Typical evaluation models ask you to evaluate attainment of knowledge, attitude, and skills separately. Unfortunately, most preceptors do not conceptualize learner performance according to these attributes. Outside the milieu of full-time educators, these concepts are somewhat foreign, and the format is not intuitive. The RIME evaluation framework avoids the somewhat artificial distinction of evaluating the individual components of medical competencies and uses a "developmental" approach instead. Each step in the RIME model represents a synthesis of knowledge, attitude, and skill that is practiced from the preclinical years of medical school through residency training. Being able to master each level, of course, depends on mastering the previous level.

Teachers who have been trained to use the RIME evaluation framework are able to obtain reliability measures (i.e., the ability to get the same result with repeated evaluations) that exceed 80% (8). A reliability measurement this high is sufficient for important evaluations, such as at the end of the rotation or year. The RIME framework also has strong predictive validity characteristics; in other words, the results predict measures of future performance, such as in an internship.

Reporter Skills

Learners who master the reporter skills can efficiently and accurately collect history and physical-examination data, can recognize normal from abnormal, and can identify and label new problems. Additionally, they are capable of communicating this information orally and in writing. Mastery of these skills is expected of all third-year students.

Interpreter Skills

Mastery of interpreter skills requires the learner to prioritize problems, to create differential diagnoses prioritized from most likely to least likely, and to follow up on and interpret results of physical findings and diagnostic tests. Acquisition of this skill marks the transition from "bystander" to active participant in patient care. Mastery of this skill level is associated with a high passing or honors grade for a third-year student and is expected of a first-year resident.

Manager Skills

Mastery of manager skills requires the learner to determine when action is necessary versus patient observation, to select the best diagnostic and therapeutic options, and to customize care according to patient circumstances and preferences. Mastery of this skill requires advanced knowledge, confidence, and judgment. This skill level is most often seen in junior and senior (second- and third-year) residents.

Educator Skills

Mastery of the educator skills requires the learner to identify knowledge gaps consistently and to develop plans for addressing these gaps. Such individuals share new knowledge with others and understand the uses and limits of evidence in the care of patients. These

skills takes drive, insight, and maturity and are most likely to charac-
terize senior residents.

❖ When and How Should the Evaluation Session Be Scheduled?

In contrast to feedback, a summative evaluation (as we have defined
it) occurs once at the end of the teaching experience. A time should
be set aside to review the evaluation with the learner before the evaluation form is returned to the sponsoring institution. Having the
learner fill out a copy of the evaluation before this meeting can be a
helpful transition into the evaluation discussion. This sets the stage for
the upcoming discussion by reminding the learner of the learning
goals and evaluation criteria. Letting the learner summarize his or her
self-assessment using the evaluation form also can provide a comfortable transition to your own observations. Additionally, self-evaluation provides an opportunity to practice the type of professional
behavior expected of physicians in the "real world."

After the learner has summarized his or her performance, you can
confirm, elaborate, or modify the self-assessment with your own
observations and conclusions. You will be surprised how accurately
learners evaluate their own performance, particularly in areas of
needed improvement. The rare learner who fails to identify important
areas of improvement may have poor insight, and this should be
brought to his or her (and the institution's) attention.

Just like when you are providing feedback, you need to be as
specific as possible in the evaluation process, citing examples of
behaviors that support your evaluation decisions. It is helpful to have
the learner sign the evaluation report at the end of the session, indicating that it was reviewed with him or her.

Fill out the institution's evaluation form as soon as you can. The
longer you wait, the more difficult it becomes to remember the
specifics of the learner's performance. In this case, you might have a
good feeling for the overall performance of the learner but will be

unable to justify your conclusions. Make a copy of the evaluation form and file it. This ensures against the evaluation being lost at the sponsoring institution and having to fill out another form. Finally, return the evaluation on time to the course director.

REFERENCES

1. **Skeff KM.** Enhancing teaching effectiveness and vitality in the ambulatory setting. *J Gen Intern Med.* 1988;3(Suppl):S26–33.
2. **McGee SR, Irby DM.** Teaching in the outpatient clinic: practical tips. *J Gen Intern Med.* 1997;12(Suppl):S34–40.
3. **Ende J.** Feedback in clinical medical education. *JAMA.* 1983;250:777–81.
4. **Cope DW, Linn LS, Leake BD, Barrett PA.** Modification of residents' behavior by preceptor feedback of patient satisfaction. *J Gen Intern Med.* 1986;1:394–8.
5. **Anderson WA, Malacrea RF.** *Giving Constructive Feedback: A Professional Development Workshop Package.* East Lansing, MI: Office of Medical Education Research and Development, College of Human Medicine, Michigan State University; 1987.
6. **Weaver MJ, Ow CL, Walker DJ, Degenhardt EF.** A questionnaire for patients' evaluations of their physicians' humanistic behaviors. *J Gen Intern Med.* 1993;8:135–9.
7. **Tamblyn R, Benaroya S, Snell L, et al.** The feasibility and value of using patient satisfaction ratings to evaluate internal medicine residents. *J Gen Intern Med.* 1994;9:149–52.
8. **Pangaro L.** A new vocabulary and other innovations for improving descriptive in-training evaluations. *Acad Med.* 1999;74:41–5.

8

Preceptor Evaluation and Teaching Improvement

❖ How Will You Be Evaluated?

In any teaching program, preceptors should be evaluated. This allows the sponsoring institution to monitor the quality of the educational program and to make improvements where they are needed. Most often, preceptors are evaluated by students or residents at the end of the rotation using a standard evaluation form (*see "Preceptor Evaluation Form" on page 131*). Although many programs attempt to get the learner to complete the preceptor's evaluation before receiving their end-of-rotation evaluation, this does not always occur. The evaluation form is often formatted to reflect the learning goals of the experience and asks to what extent you were able to help the learner achieve those goals. This process is no different than that used for full-time faculty at medical schools and residency programs, yet it is not always a comfortable experience.

At some point, a summary of all your learners' evaluations will be returned to you. This often takes place after a large number of learners have rotated through your office to increase the sample size and, therefore, the reliability of the process. Most institutions will summarize the scores of the learners and provide a mean score for each category on the evaluation form. Provided that the institution's program is large enough, comparison data consisting of mean scores derived from other preceptor evaluations will be provided. This will allow you to compare your performance against your peers. Written comments from the learners usually are collected for your review. Depending on the policy of the sponsoring institution, the authors of the comments on the evaluation form may or may not be identified.

Despite the fact you have sacrificed time and, sometimes, income to be a preceptor, the evaluations will not always reflect this effort. Therefore, it is important to be philosophical about the evaluations and to recognize that you will never be able to please everyone; however, the evaluations can provide you with important information about the experience. For example, you may use the evaluations to modify your office experience to better help the learners achieve the stated program goals and to reinforce the experiences that were well received and in accordance with the institution's expectations. You may seek help from the institution for advice if parts of your experience fall short of expectations. Most institutions are willing to provide site visits and explore ways to improve the experience.

❖ How Can You Improve Your Teaching?

In the context of professional practice, reflection has been shown to be key in the educational experiences of both learners and teachers. Teachers must be able to reflect on their instruction if they are to identify ways of improving it (1,2). Reflection can occur in all stages of the teaching process, from planning to after a learner has moved on. Anticipatory reflection includes organizing and preparing for a learning session, selecting teaching strategies, and tailoring the teaching to the needs of the learner. Good teaching requires that you consider the needs and interests of learners and adapt the teaching to meet learners' needs (to the extent that is possible when teaching "on the run").

Reflection during the teaching process involves making necessary adjustments to each changing teaching situation. Inflexibility on the part of the teacher at this stage can result in poor teaching performance. An example of inflexibility is continuing to explain the reasons for selecting one therapy over another when it is obvious that the learner is unclear about the basic disease process. The preceptor who can, through reflection, recognize a learner's difficulty, drop the discussion of therapy, and substitute one about disease mechanism and natural history is more likely to be successful.

For many preceptors, reflection after teaching provides the impetus for change and improvement. Assessing what went well and what went wrong are key steps in this self-evaluation process. Excellent preceptors use this information to make their teaching more effective and relevant for the learner. Less effective teachers never change or even consider the need to change.

Teaching failures *will* occur; they are an integral part of the process. However, when confronted with failure, there are several things you can do. First, be realistic; even the best of teachers have bad days when nothing seems to work. Second, keep your "antennae" out to recognize the parts that were and were not successful. If you are lucky, you can ask for and receive useful feedback; however, this often will not occur, so you must personally observe what engages the learner and adjust your teaching accordingly (2).

❖ Workshops, Courses, Peer Site Visits, and Additional Resources

Faculty-development courses are traditional methods of improving the teaching skills of both full-time and community preceptors. Usually, the course is scheduled over a two- or three-day period, but many formats can be designed to accommodate community physicians. Perceptions of these courses are typically positive, and the benefit of attending often exceeds the participants' expectations—they report improvement in their ability to foster a constructive learning climate, to communicate goals, to provide feedback, and to teach overall (3).

Peer site visits have been used successfully to improve teaching. Participants in such visits indicate that these provide a unique and helpful opportunity for reflective discussion. Others see site visits as opportunities to validate and affirm their approaches to teaching and to foster a strong sense of collegiality (4).

Other resources to improve teaching skills can be found on the Internet or are available on CD-ROM or videotape. If you are interested in these resources, you can contact the American College of Physicians-American Society of Internal Medicine via the Internet at http://www.acponline.org/cme/cbt or by calling 800-523-1546, ext. 2615.

REFERENCES

1. **Skeff KM, Bowen JL, Irby DM.** Protecting time for teaching in the ambulatory care setting. *Acad Med.* 1997;72:694–7.
2. **Pinsky LE, Irby DM.** "If at first you don't succeed": using failure to improve teaching. *Acad Med.* 1997;72:973–6.
3. **Skeff KM, Stratos GA, Bergen MR, et al.** Regional teaching improvement programs for community-based teachers. *Am J Med.* 1999;106:76–80.
4. **Bing-You RG, Renfrew RA, Hampton SH.** Faculty development of community-based preceptors through a collegial site-visit program. *Teach Learn Med.* 1999;11:100–4.

APPENDIX A

Quick Tips for Preceptors

❖ Before the Learner Arrives Preparatory Checklist
See "Before the Learner Arrives" on page 19.

One Week Before the Learner Arrives
❑ Review the institution's learning goals and objectives

❑ Review the institution's orientation materials

❑ Review the student's information or application (if available)

❑ Have a reliable number for the institution's contact person in case of problems

❑ Have staff confirm the dates and times of the instruction in your office with the sponsoring institution

❑ Send any information the learner should know about the practice to the sponsoring institution for distribution to the learner

❑ Schedule a 30-minute orientation for the learner

❑ Schedule time at the end of the experience for learner evaluation and feedback

❑ Consider making a brochure or handout for patients about the learner (*see "Biography of a Resident Physician" on page 120*)

❑ Consider altering your schedule for the precepting experience (*see "Patient Scheduling" on page 25*)

Two to Three Days Before the Learner Arrives
❑ Remind staff and partners of the impending arrival of the learner

❑ Distribute copy of the learner's application or personal information (if available) to staff and partners

❑ Brief the staff on the learner's responsibilities

❑ Review with the staff their role with the learner

❑ Coach the staff on how to present the learner to patients

❑ Identify a parking place for the learner

❑ Identify a workspace for the learner

❑ Equip workspace with needed references, paper, and writing utensils

❑ Gather forms (e.g., laboratory, physical therapy, radiology, consultation) for learner orientation

❑ Generate list of staff, their office locations, and a short description of their responsibilities (save in file)

❑ Make copies of patient notices about the learner for reception area (*see "Patient Notice for Students in the Office" and "Patient Notice for Residents in the Office" on pages 118 and 119*)

❑ Make a list of what to cover during learner orientation (save in file; *see "When the Learner Arrives Orientation Checklist" on page 96*)

❑ If the learner will dictate notes, prepare instructions (save in file)

❖ When the Learner Arrives Orientation Checklist

See "When the Learner Arrives" on page 22.

❑ Post notices in the reception area about the learner

❑ Have the receptionist inform patients about the learner

❑ Review with the learner the institution's learning goals and objectives

❑ Review the "Clinical Skills Inventory" with learner (*see "Previous Experiences" on page 22*)

❑ Review the learner's expectations for this experience

❑ Review your expectations for the experience

❑ Consider signing a learning contract with learner (*see "Learner Contract" on page 116*)

❑ Review working hours

❑ Review days off

❑ Review potential schedule conflicts and attempt to resolve them

❑ Review how to contact office in case of personal emergency or unanticipated schedule conflict

❑ Review office rules and policies (e.g., parking, dress code, meals, telephone and computer use)

❑ Orient the learner to his or her personal workspace

❑ Review contents of examination room and where equipment, supplies, and forms are located

❑ Introduce learner to staff (including their responsibilities) and to partners

❑ Review when and how teaching will occur

❑ Review when and how feedback will be provided

❑ Review scheduling and which patients the learner will see

❑ Review how much time should be spent with patients

❑ Review what parts of examination should and should not be done in your absence

❑ Review how to organize the learner's time with the patient and you (*see "Strategies for Organizing the Office Visit" on page 37*)

❑ Review how you want patients presented to you (*see "Patient Presentation Format for Learners" on page 126*)
❑ Review how you want notes written or dictated
❑ Review which clinical tests are performed in the office
❑ Review how to order imaging studies and other diagnostic tests
❑ Review how to schedule a consultation
❑ Review how to schedule a follow-up appointment
❑ Review where to retrieve patient education materials
❑ Review how to retrieve test results
❑ Review how to request a patient chart
❑ Review when the final evaluation will take place
❑ Review how to handle an office emergency (e.g., cardiac arrest)

❖ When the Patients Arrive Checklist

See "When the Patients Arrive" on page 28.

❑ Have the receptionist inform patients that you have a learner in the office today

❑ Distribute brochure or handout about the learner to patients, if available (*see "Biography of a Resident Physician" on page 120*)

❑ Ask the patient's permission before bringing a learner into the examination room

   ▶ Couch your request positively, e.g., "I have a medical student/resident working with me today. If it's okay with you, I'd like him/her to talk to you and examine you first. I will come in and see you afterwards."

❑ If you teach frequently, inform new patients that you work with learners

❑ Have the office staff inform you about any positive or negative feedback from the patients about the learner

❑ Consider measuring your patients' satisfaction with the learner by using the *"Patient Satisfaction Form" on page 130*

❖ Summary of the Learning Experience

❑ Expose the learner to all the things you do as a physician and as a member of the community
  ► How you relate to other specialists and medical professionals
  ► How you keep up on medical knowledge
  ► What you do in the hospital and in other settings
  ► Your participation in professional organizations
  ► Your civic and community activities

❑ Require novice learners to observe you with selected patients performing various skills
  ► Taking a focused history
  ► Performing part of an examination
  ► Performing a procedure
  ► Counseling a patient

❑ Provide opportunities for the learner to see patients first (alone)
  ► Take the history
  ► Perform the examination
  ► Form their own impressions about diagnosis
  ► Generate a management plan
  ► Report to you
  ► Write the orders
  ► Write the prescription
  ► Arrange for follow-up

❑ Organize the visit for the learner (see "Tools To Help Organize the Patient Visit" on page 124)
  ► "Prime" the learner by providing pertinent patient-specific background information, e.g., "Mrs. Jones is a healthy 28-year-old woman and is here for her yearly examination. At her age, what are the important screening issues to be covered?"
  ► "Frame" the visit by focusing on what should be accomplished at this visit and how long it should take, e.g., "This patient has several problems, but today I'd like you to focus on the

patient's care of her diabetes. Spend 15 minutes taking the history and then come find me."

❑ Familiarize yourself with the common models of case-based learning (*see Chapter 5*)
  ▶ Microskills model
  ▶ "Aunt Minnie" model
  ▶ Modeling Problem Solving
  ▶ The One-Minute Observation
  ▶ Learner-Centered Precepting
❑ Set "mini-goals"
❑ Consider strategies to improve teaching efficiency (*see Chapter 6*)
  ▶ Consider a wave schedule (*see "Patient Scheduling" on page 25 and "The Wave Schedule" on pages 26 and 128*)
  ▶ Have the learner present the case in front of the patient in the examination room
  ▶ Encourage collaborative examinations
  ▶ Use the technique of active observation (*see "Active Observation" on page 68 and "Summary of Active Observation" on page 106*), e.g., "Let's counsel this patient about quitting smoking. Watch my approach. I'd like you to review this [brief chapter or paper] and try to counsel the next patient with this problem."
  ▶ Expose the learner to educational experiences beyond patient care
  ▶ Expose the learner to service-based education
  ▶ Have the learner keep notes of questions to be discussed at the end of the day
  ▶ Have the learner engage in "Self-Directed (Independent) Learning" (*see page 70 and "Summary of Self-Directed [Independent] Learning" on page 107*)
❑ Ending the day
  ▶ Meet with the learner to discuss unanswered questions or concerns
  ▶ Encourage independent learning by assigning "homework"
  ▶ Follow up with learner on any "homework" assignments
  ▶ Consider using the "Educational Prescription Form" (*see page 129*)
❑ Feedback and evaluation (*see Chapter 7*)

- ▶ Provide frequent, timely feedback
- ▶ Base evaluation on evidence
- ▶ Consider using the "RIME Evaluation Framework" (*see page 83 and "Summary of RIME Evaluation Framework" on page 111*)

❖ Summary of the Microskills Model for Precepting

See "The Microskills Model" on page 44.

❑ Get a commitment
  ▶ Ask the learner to commit to some decision or plan of action, e.g., "What do you think is going on with this patient?"
❑ Probe for supporting evidence
  ▶ Ask the learner for the evidence that supports the commitment, e.g., "What were the major findings that led you to that diagnosis?", "Why did you choose medication X rather than medication Y?"
❑ Teach general rules
  ▶ Teaching is more memorable and more easily transferable to other cases when it is offered as a general rule rather than as a patient-specific plan, e.g., "In a young patient with mechanical low back pain, an X-ray is not needed initially."
❑ Reinforce what was done right
  ▶ Provide positive, explicit, behavior-specific feedback, e.g., "You were very empathic with that patient, and she responded by providing important information in the history."
  ▶ Positive feedback is not general praise, e.g., "You did a good job with that last patient."
❑ Correct mistakes
  ▶ Attempt to frame the mistake as being "not the best" rather than "bad" or "wrong."
  ▶ Provide specific guidance on improvement, e.g., "You might be more successful next time this happens if you try…"

❖ Summary of the "Aunt Minnie" Model of Precepting

See "The 'Aunt Minnie' Model" on page 53.

❏ Have the learner collect data from the patient
   ▶ If the patient problem is straightforward, the learner informs the preceptor that he or she has an "Aunt Minnie" case
   ▶ If the patient problem is not straightforward, then either the preceptor uses the microskills or other case-based teaching model
❏ The learner presents only the chief complaint and probable diagnosis (30 seconds)
❏ Have the learner write the note
❏ Examine the patient without the learner present
❏ Provide feedback to the learner by doing one of the following:
   ▶ Confirm the diagnosis
   ▶ Provide the correct diagnosis (1–5 minutes)
❏ Review the learner's written note

❖ Summary of the One-Minute Observation

See "The One-Minute Observation" on page 56.

❏ Explain the purpose of the observation to the learner
❏ Explain how the observation will occur
❏ Select one skill for observation
❏ Inform the patient of what will take place
❏ Observe for a brief period of time without interrupting
❏ Leave the room and have the learner join you when finished with the patient
❏ Provide immediate feedback on what you observed
❏ Use the information gained to plan your teaching
❏ Repeat the process observing other skills
❏ Evaluate the learner's skills over time, using multiple, brief periods of observation

❖ Summary of Learner-Centered Precepting

See "Learner-Centered Precepting" on page 57.

Identification

☐ Learner presents patient
  ▶ Gives name and age
  ▶ Specifies whether the patient is new or a return
  ▶ Details chief complaint
  ▶ Identifies teaching need, e.g., "My question is, should Mrs. Smith have an insulin pump?"

Information

☐ Learner presents patient data, diagnosis, and plan
  ▶ Gives concise history
  ▶ Details pertinent examination findings
  ▶ Determines most likely diagnosis
  ▶ Develops treatment plan

Issues

☐ Learner formulates specific questions needed to care for patient
  ▶ Verification of findings
  ▶ Content (knowledge) information
  ▶ Logistical information

❖ Summary of Active Observation

See "Active Observation" on page 68.

❑ Explain the rationale for the observation, e.g., "You should watch me do this because you need help with cardiac auscultation"

❑ Tell the learner what to observe, e.g., "Notice how I listen to the patient's heart in several positions and use both the bell and diaphragm."

❑ Ask the learner should review with you what was observed, e.g., "Tell me how I examined the heart"

❑ Tell the learner to practice the skill just demonstrated, e.g., "When you see the next patient, I want you to practice cardiac auscultation"

❑ Give feedback to the learner on how he or she performed the skill

❑ *Important Point:* Active observation is not simply "shadowing"; it should be performed with well-defined learner goals and accountabilities

❖ Summary of Self-Directed (Independent) Learning

See "Self-Directed (Independent) Learning" on page 70.

Identify the Need

❑ After hearing the patient presentation (or at the end of the session), have the learner either identify his or her learning question or prompt him or her by asking
  ▶ "Based on the patients you saw today, what are your questions?"
  ▶ "What is the one thing you would like to learn more about?"
  ▶ "What troubled you today?"
  ▶ "What might you improve?"

Make an Assignment

❑ Ask the learner to formulate the question
❑ Ask the learner to research the answer to the question
❑ Specify a time for the learner to report back to you with the results of the research

Identify Potential Resources

❑ Textbooks (print and electronic)
❑ MEDLINE or other databases
❑ Journal articles
❑ Consultants

"Close the Loop"

❑ The learner reports back on what was found
  ▶ Gives an oral presentation
  ▶ Submits a written outline
  ▶ Incorporates it into a patient write-up or assessment
❑ Consider using the "Educational Prescription Form" (*see page 129*) to facilitate the learning

❖ Summary of Feedback

See "What Are Some Effective Methods of Learner Feedback?" on page 75.

❏ Feedback should be ongoing and frequent
  ▶ The most common complaint of learners is that nobody tells them how they are doing
❏ Give the feedback as soon as possible after a critical incident
❏ Use notes to help you recall the points you wish to make
❏ Use the "feedback sandwich"
❏ Describe the observed behavior
❏ Be as specific as possible
❏ End the feedback with detailed instructions for improvement
❏ Follow up with positive feedback and praise the learner when improvement occurs

Constructive Feedback Has Several Identifiable Qualities

CONSTRUCTIVE FEEDBACK

Quality	*Comment*	*Good Example*	*Poor Example*
Descriptive, not evaluative	Describes the behavior you observe without attributing value to it	"You did not make eye contact with the last patient during the interview"	"You are not interested in patient care" "Your personality is not suitable for a physician"
Specific, not general	Identifies the precise behavior you wish to highlight, avoiding generalities	"You were able to convey empathy and understanding during the interview"	"You did a good job" "You could have done better"
Focused on issues the learner can control	Provides tips on how to improve	"When taking the history, speak slower and check for understanding"	"My patients cannot understand you because of your accent"
Well timed	Makes feedback an expectation, not an exception	When it is provided regularly throughout the learning experience and as close as possible to the event that brought about the feedback	When it is provided only at the end of the rotation
Limited in amount	Make the message memorable	When it focuses on a single, important message	When the learner is overwhelmed with information
Addresses learner goals	Refers back to the learner contract (*see "Expectations" on page 22 and "Learner Contract" on page 116*) or other information gathered during the orientation	When it addresses goals that were identified by the learner at the beginning of the office experience	When the learner's goals are ignored

❖ Summary of Evaluation

See "What Are Some Effective Methods of Learner Evaluation?" on page 78.

❑ Summative evaluation occurs at the end of instruction
  ▶ Review the learner's past performance
  ▶ Base your review on the sponsoring institution's evaluation criteria
❑ The final evaluation should never be a surprise to the learner
  ▶ Avoid surprise by providing specific feedback periodically throughout the precepting experience
❑ Consider referring to the "RIME Evaluation Framework" (*see page 83 and "Summary of RIME Evaluation Framework" on page 111*) before evaluating the learner
  ▶ Base the evaluation on systematic, first-hand observations of the learner's performance
❑ Emphasize changes in behavior and performance that will lead to the desired competencies
❑ Deliver the evaluation in oral and written forms
❑ Make a copy of your evaluation and file it
❑ Return the written evaluation to the sponsoring institution on time
❑ Avoid rating errors when filling out the written evaluation form
  ▶ *The "halo/horn" effect:* Basing your evaluation on reports of previous performance
  ▶ *Restriction of range:* Using the same rating for all components of the evaluation, rather than rating each individually
  ▶ *Rating nonperformance attributes:* Taking into consideration behavior attributes when rating nonbehavioral qualities
❑ Schedule time for the evaluation when you will not be interrupted or hurried
❑ Begin the evaluation by having the learner perform a self-assessment
❑ Consider having the learner fill out a copy of the final evaluation form provided by the institution before your meeting
❑ Use the learner's self-evaluation to begin the discussion of your own observations

❖ Summary of the RIME Evaluation Framework

See "The RIME Evaluation Framework" on page 83.

Reporter

❑ One who can efficiently and accurately collect patient data

❑ One who can recognize normal from abnormal

❑ One who can identify and label new problems

❑ One who can communicate collected data orally and in writing

Interpreter

❑ One who can prioritize problems

❑ One who can follow up and interpret abnormal findings and tests

❑ One who can create a differential diagnosis

❑ One who can prioritize a differential diagnosis

Manager

❑ One who can determine when action is necessary

❑ One who can choose the most appropriate diagnostic test

❑ One who can choose the most appropriate management strategy

❑ One who can customize a plan according to patient circumstances and preferences

Educator

❑ One who can identify knowledge gaps and develop plans to address them

❑ One who can share new knowledge with others

❑ One who can understand the use and limits of evidence in the care of patients

APPENDIX B

Tools for Preceptors

❖ Clinical Skills Inventory

To be filled out by the learner at or before the orientation.
See "When the Learner Arrives" on page 22.

Student Name _____

Part I. To help your preceptor improve your clinical skills, please indicate your experience by checking the appropriate box.

Physical Examination	No Experience	Some Experience	Much Experience
1. Adolescent	❑	❑	❑
2. Complete adult	❑	❑	❑
3. System focused	❑	❑	❑
4. Breast	❑	❑	❑
5. Pelvic	❑	❑	❑
6. Rectal	❑	❑	❑
7. Prostate	❑	❑	❑
8. Cardiovascular	❑	❑	❑
9. Abdominal	❑	❑	❑
10. Pulmonary	❑	❑	❑
11. Musculoskeletal	❑	❑	❑

Part II. Are there other areas in which you feel that you need specific instruction? Please check the appropriate boxes.

Procedures	No Experience	Some Experience	Much Experience
1. Electrocardiogram interpretation	❑	❑	❑
2. Flexible sigmoidoscopy	❑	❑	❑
3. Gram stain interpretation	❑	❑	❑
4. Joint aspiration/injection	❑	❑	❑
5. KOH (skin)	❑	❑	❑
6. Soft-tissue trigger injection	❑	❑	❑
7. Pap smear	❑	❑	❑
8. Testing stool for blood	❑	❑	❑
9. Throat culture	❑	❑	❑
10. Urinalysis (dip stick)	❑	❑	❑
11. Urinalysis (microscopic)	❑	❑	❑
12. Wet mount/vaginal	❑	❑	❑
13. Skin biopsy	❑	❑	❑

Part III. Are there other areas in which you feel that you need specific instruction?

_____

_____

_____

_____

_____

❖ Learner Contract

To be given to the learner at the time of orientation.
See "When the Learner Arrives" on page 22.

Student Name _____

Preceptor Name _____

Part I. Student's Goals

List the three most important goals you have for this preceptorship.

1. _____
2. _____
3. _____

List specific strategies you suggest for accomplishing these goals.

_____

_____

_____

_____

Part II. Preceptor's Goals

List the three most important areas on which you believe the student should focus:

1. _____
2. _____
3. _____

List strategies you suggest for addressing these areas:

_____

_____

_____

_____

Part III. Summary
Performance goals and expectations are:

_____

_____

_____

_____

Student Name _____ **Date** _____

Preceptor Name _____ **Date** _____

❖ Patient Notice for Students in the Office

See "When the Learner Arrives" on page 22.

To our patients:

Our office is pleased to be participating in a supervised clinical learning program for medical students.

This type of education and training in places not associated with a medical school or hospital helps ensure that our future physicians will have the knowledge and experience they'll need for the "real world" of medical practice.

Your support of this program is helping train excellent doctors for the future.

Thank you.

❖ Patient Notice for Residents in the Office

See "When the Learner Arrives" on page 22.

To our patients:

Our office is pleased to be participating in a supervised clinical learn-ing program for internal medicine residents (doctors who are training to be specialists in adult medicine).

This type of education and training in places not associated with a medical school or hospital helps ensure that our future physicians will have the knowledge and experience they'll need for the "real world" of medical practice.

Your support of this program is helping us train excellent doctors for the future.

Thank you.

❖ Biography of a Resident Physician

To be made available in the office reception area.
See "When the Patients Arrive" on page 28.

New Resident Bio: Katie Smith, MD

I grew up in Flint, Michigan, and graduated from Michigan State University where I studied art history and studio art. After receiving a fellowship in art history at the University of Michigan, I had the opportunity to live and study in Paris. After six months, however, I decided to return home to pursue a career in medicine, a decision that was strongly influenced by my father's illness.

I am a graduate of Michigan State University College of Human Medicine and now live in Grand Rapids, with my husband, Richard, and son, Bart. I am specializing in internal medicine and hope to practice here in Grand Rapids. My interests include traveling, cooking, skiing, and snorkeling.

❖ Instructions To Help Organize the Patient Visit

See "Strategies for Organizing the Office Visit" in on page 37.

Instructions for Students and Residents

Welcome to our office. We hope that you find providing care for patients in an office setting as enjoyable and as stimulating as we do. You will discover that outpatient care requires different skills from those you have learned practicing hospital medicine. The following paragraphs illustrate a few tips to help you begin.

A good patient visit requires effective organization of your time with the patient. Before all visits, mentally organize the encounter, including the time you spend with the patient. For return patients, remind yourself of the visit goal. You may want to review a visit plan with the preceptor before seeing the patient.

Begin the visit by setting mutual expectations about the agenda and the allotted time. Determine the patient's agenda for the visit with the question, "What concerns do you have today?" Limit the number of problems to two or three so they can be addressed within the allotted time. Prioritize problems by their severity, urgency, or importance to the patient, as appropriate. For return visits, state your agenda first, then ask for the patient's expectations. For example, you might say, "Mr. Smith, we have 20 minutes today. I'd like to follow up on your high blood pressure. Is there anything else you want to discuss?" If your and the patient's expectations do not match, negotiate how you are going to spend the time by saying something like, "That sounds like more than we will have time to discuss today. What two things are most important or pressing for you? We can address those issues today and set up another appointment to begin to address the others." This approach will satisfy most patients.

Patients appreciate when they know you are listening and including them in the planning. Determine what the patient thinks is going on and what they want done by asking, "What do *you* think is causing this? What do *you* think should be done?"

Early into the encounter, develop a favored initial hypothesis and consider its supporting evidence. Mentally create a weighted differential diagnosis and estimate the probability (low, medium, or high) of each. Consider the impact of not making an unlikely but important diagnosis emergently. For example, "In this patient, do I need to rule out ischemic heart disease as the cause of the chest pain even though it sounds like acid reflux?" Establish an initial focused action for each problem, including history, focused physical examination, tests, and treatment.

Office presentations are different from those performed in hospital wards. Many students and residents are taught to present as completely as possible, demonstrating their thoroughness. Other expectations include discussing all the patient's medical issues. Although these approaches are appropriate in some settings, the focus and time limitations in the office necessitate a different approach. The goals in the ambulatory setting are to emphasize the information needed for the patient's care *at this time* and to present as a concise summary to the preceptor as possible. The office presentation should begin with the patient identification, including whether her or she is a new or return patient and if the problem is acute or chronic. Next, give a statement of what questions *you* have as a result of your interaction with the patient. For example, "I am seeing a long-term patient of yours. He is 65 years old and was last seen three months ago for a cough that we attributed to a URI. He returns today because the cough persists. I have questions about where to go in his evaluation." Two other examples of prefacing your presentation with learning questions that need to be answered include: "I am seeing a 25-year-old woman, a new patient, who came in to establish care without any specific complaints. I had some questions about my findings on skin examination" and "Mr. Smith is a 40-year-old patient of yours who is here for pain medication for a migraine. I have questions about how to prescribe this medication for migraine headaches."

The patient identification and learner question is followed by a concise history of the presenting problems and a report of the focused physical examination. Do not report everything you know about the patient, only the pertinent positive and negative findings. (*Note:* You should know everything about the patient but you do not need tell the preceptor everything you know.) State your most likely diagnosis with brief supporting evidence. Include any diagnoses that you would not want to miss (e.g., worst-case scenarios) and their likelihood. Present your plan with brief supporting evidence. State it as best you can, recognizing that parts may hinge on the question(s) you need answered. Discuss your question and plan with the preceptor. Prepare the follow-up.

Patient education should be concise and clear enough that the patient can go home and explain to a friend or family member "what the doctor said." Assess the patient's level of understanding by asking questions, for example, "I think your skin rash is most likely due to psoriasis. Have you heard of psoriasis? What do you know about psoriasis?" Based on the patient's response, direct your education accordingly. Avoid the use of medical jargon (e.g., use "rash" instead of "lesions").

If the patient brings up a problem at the end of the visit ("I forgot to mention my back pain"), do not despair. Quickly assess and triage the situation to an immediate evaluation versus following up with it at the next visit. In assessing the seriousness of the condition, it may be helpful to consider why the patient did not mention it earlier. Was it because he or she is afraid of its seriousness, is simply being complete, or is truly just remembering it? Also, the patient may not want closure and is not ready for you to leave. Ask the preceptor for help if you are unsure if a problem needs to be evaluated emergently.

❖ Tools To Help the Learner Organize the Patient Visit

What?—The Patient's Agenda
"What should we talk about today?"

Problem 1	Problem 2	Problem 3

Why?—The Patient's Attribution
"What do you think is causing this? What do you think should be done?"

Problem 1	Problem 2	Problem 3

Why?—The Favored Initial Hypothesis

Problem 1	Problem 2	Problem 3
Supporting Evidence	Supporting Evidence	Supporting Evidence

What Else?—The Differential Diagnosis

Estimate probability "[P]" as being "L" (low), "M" (medium), or "H" (high)

Problem 1	Problem 2	Problem 3
[P]=	[P]=	[P]=
[P]=	[P]=	[P]=
[P]=	[P]=	[P]=

What Now?—Initial Focused Actions

Problem 1	Problem 2	Problem 3
History:	History:	History:
Exam:	Exam:	Exam:
Tests:	Tests:	Tests:
Therapy:	Therapy:	Therapy:

❖ Patient Presentation Format for Learners

See "Strategies for Organizing the Office Visit" on page 37.

Identifying Data and Chief Complaint
❑ Patient name
❑ Age
❑ New or return visit (last seen _____)
❑ Questions from the last visit that need to be addressed
❑ New questions for today

Questions Needing Answers (General)
❑ Diagnostic uncertainty
❑ History to ask
❑ Pertinent examination to perform
❑ Verify examination findings
❑ Further evaluation
❑ Treatment
❑ Follow-up
❑ Social services

Concise History of Present Illness
❑ Include only pertinent positive and negative findings
❑ History
❑ Past medical history
❑ Social history
❑ Family history

Concise Physical Examination
❑ Only pertinent positive and negative findings
❑ Most likely diagnosis
❑ Provide brief supporting evidence
❑ Estimate likelihood
❑ Include any "wouldn't-want-to-miss" diagnoses
❑ Your plan may depend on answers to your questions

Questions Needing Answers (Specific)

❑ Diagnostic questions
❑ Treatment plan
❑ Plans for follow-up

❖ The Wave Schedule

See "Patient Scheduling" on page 25.

WAVE SCHEDULE

Time (AM)	Original Physician Schedule	Learner Wave Schedule	Physician Wave Schedule
8:00–8:20	Patient A	Patient A	Patient B
8:20–8:40	Patient B	Patient A	Patient A
840–9:00	Patient C	Writes note	Patient C
9:00–9:20	Patient D	Patient D	Patient E
9:20–9:40	Patient E	Patient D	Patient D
9:40–10:00	Patient F	Writes note	Patient F
10:00–10:20	Patient G	Patient G	Patient H
10:20–10:40	Patient H	Patient G	Patient G
10:40–11:00	Patient I	Writes note	Patient I
11:00–11:20	Patient J	Patient J	Patient K
11:20–11:40	Patient K	Patient J	Patient J
11:40–Noon	Patient L	Writes note	Patient L

▶ This model allows physicians to see the same number of patients promptly with a learner present

▶ The wave schedule can be more intense for advanced learners

▶ The wave schedule can be less intense for the novice learner

▶ This model is easily adaptable to schedules of any appointment length, provided that the slots are of equal length

❖ Educational Prescription Form

See "Self-Directed (Indedpendent) Learning" on page 70.

Date and place to be filled _____

Patient's problem _____

_____

_____

_____

_____

Educational tasks to be completed before the session

Learner: _____

Task: _____

_____

Presentation will cover:

▶ How you found what you found
▶ What you found
▶ The validity and applicability of what you found
▶ How what you found will alter your management of the patient
▶ How well you think you did in filling this educational prescription

❖ Patient Satisfaction Form

See "What Are Some Effective Methods of Learner Evaluation?" on page 78.

This Doctor:	Strongly Disagree				Strongly Agree
Follows through on problems	1	2	3	4	5
Is truthful and honest with me without avoiding the issues	1	2	3	4	5
Is in a hurry	1	2	3	4	5
Expresses concern for my feelings and needs, not just my physical status	1	2	3	4	5
Comforts or reassures me and my family	1	2	3	4	5
Asks me how I am doing	1	2	3	4	5
Keeps his or her promises to me	1	2	3	4	5
Pays attention to concerns and requests that I feel are important	1	2	3	4	5
Explains and clarifies information for me	1	2	3	4	5
Answers my questions	1	2	3	4	5
Makes uncaring remarks or does things I find offensive	1	2	3	4	5
Discusses the options for my treatment	1	2	3	4	5
Uses terms that I can understand	1	2	3	4	5
Includes me in decisions and choices about my care	1	2	3	4	5
Arranges for adequate privacy when examining or talking with me	1	2	3	4	5
Has a neat, clean, well-groomed appearance	1	2	3	4	5
Is short-tempered or abrupt with my family or me	1	2	3	4	5
Does not rush or spend too little time with me	1	2	3	4	5
Asks if I need anything or what he or she can do for me	1	2	3	4	5
Asks how I want to be addressed, then greets me in that way	1	2	3	4	5
Seems knowledgeable and concerned about my case and me	1	2	3	4	5
Asks questions about my symptoms	1	2	3	4	5
Treats me in too intimate or personal a manner	1	2	3	4	5
Asks me how I feel about my problems	1	2	3	4	5

Republished with permission from Weaver MJ, Ow CL, Walker DJ, Degenhardt EF. A questionnaire for patients' evaluations of their physicians humanistic behaviors. *J Gen Intern Med.* 1993;8:135–9.

❖ Preceptor Evaluation Form

See "How Will You Be Evaluated?" on page 89.

Student Name _____

Preceptor Name _____

School or Program Sponsor _____

Date _____

General Information	*Yes*	*No*
1. Did you feel that your preceptor's practice gave you adequate exposure to general internal medicine?	❑	❑
2. Which of the following learner resources were available to you:		
a. Reference library	❑	❑
b. Personal computer	❑	❑
c. Audio-visual learning materials	❑	❑
d. Self-instructional materials	❑	❑

List materials not available that you feel would have been useful: _____

_____

	Yes	No
3. Did you routinely round with your preceptor in a hospital setting?	❑	❑
4. How many patients did you have contact with per half-day session? _____		
5. What was the degree of your responsibility concerning patient care? ❑ Too much ❑ Too little ❑ Appropriate		
6. How would you rate your level of supervision by the preceptor? ❑ Too much ❑ Too little ❑ Appropriate		
7. Would you recommend this experience to other students?	❑	❑
8. Would you recommend your preceptor to other students?	❑	❑
9. Did you achieve your educational objectives?	❑	❑

Please comment: _____

_____

	Yes	No
10. Were your preceptor's activities consistent with your educational goals?	❑	❑
11. Did your preceptor give you constructive feedback about your performance?	❑	❑
12. Did your preceptor allow time for teaching-learning sessions (questions and answers)?	❑	❑
13. Did your preceptor take time to review patient medical records?	❑	❑
14. Did your preceptor take time to review patient treatment?	❑	❑
15. Did your preceptor check the accuracy of your history taking?	❑	❑

continued

16. What additional comments do you have?

_____

_____

_____

17. What suggestions do you have that would increase interest in and/or improve this program?

_____

_____

_____

APPENDIX C

Resources for Preceptors

❖ Instructional Video for Office-Based Teaching

Available for a modest cost, *ACP-ASIM Teaching in the Ambulatory Setting* is an instructional video on office-based teaching that may be viewed by individuals or as part of a group faculty-development program. It runs approximately 20 minutes and comes with a companion text. Each of nine different teaching scenes (*see table below*) illustrates a different teaching strategy or problem described in this book.

CONTENT OF THE *ACP-ASIM TEACHING IN THE AMBULATORY SETTING*

Scene	Title	Content
1	Orientation/Setting Goals and Expectations	Preceptor finds out more about the learner and his or her expectations; learner is taught about the process, expectations, and office procedures
2	Student with Poor Ability or Knowledge I	Preceptor fails to get learner to commit, takes over case, but provides a good example of "modeling"
3	Student with Poor Ability or Knowledge II	Preceptor gives "destructive feedback" followed by a lecture
4	Student with Poor Ability or Knowledge III	Preceptor gets learner to commit and probes for supporting evidence
5	Student with Incomplete Database	Preceptor diagnoses cause of poor performance and proceeds to "prime the student" for the subsequent encounter
6	Student with Poor Management Plan	Preceptor recognizes a learning problem through questioning; he then gives a "feedback sandwich" and an independent study assignment
7	Student with Unprofessional Behavior	Preceptor identifies unprofessional attitudes and deals with them
8	Student Who Performs Well	Preceptor demonstrates use of the hypothetical questioning technique
9	Student Who Knows More Than the Preceptor	Learner demonstrates more knowledge in an area than the preceptor, prompting the question of how to respond and the issue of intellectual honesty

For more information about the video, call 800-523-1546, ext. 2614. To order, call 800-523-1546, ext. 2600, and request product #190400100.

❖ ACP-ASIM Awards Program

Community-Based Teaching Participation Award

To support community-based teaching physicians, ACP-ASIM offers a Teaching Participation Award. This handsome, individualized certificate is intended for prominent display in the practitioner's office. Precepting internists who have been active in office-based teaching for at least two years during a three-year period and who are nominated by a community-based teaching administrator are eligible for the award. The certificate is awarded only once to an individual preceptor. Contact the Education and Career Development Department for applications (800-523-1546, ext. 2614) or download the application from the ACP-ASIM Web site at http://www.acponline.org/cme/cbt.

Community-Based Teaching Excellence in Teaching Award

The Community-Based Teaching Excellence in Teaching Award requires involvement in office-based teaching for seven out of 10 years, with at least three years at the same sponsoring institution and an average of 50 hours of direct trainee contact during those years. In addition to the time requirement, the internist also must meet certain measures of teaching excellence defined in the application. A number of measures of teaching excellence are outlined in the award criteria to accommodate the many different ways sponsoring institutions recognize teaching excellence. As with the Community-Based Teaching Participation Award, the Excellence in Teaching Award is reserved for internal medicine physicians and awarded only once to each individual. Contact the Education and Career Development Department for applications (800-523-1546, ext. 2614) or download the application from the ACP-ASIM Web site at http://www.acponline.org/cme/cbt.

❖ Commonly Offered Rewards for Precepting

See "What Are the Most Commonly Offered Rewards for Community-Based Teaching?" on page 8.

Enhanced Capitation

One potential economic benefit is a higher capitation rate for participating physicians negotiated on their behalf by the training institution. Some programs have negotiated 1% increases (Grayson MS et al. Promoting institutional change to encourage primary care. Acad Med. 1999;74:S9–15).

CME Credits for Community-Based Teaching

Although most teaching programs do not qualify for category 1 CME credits, category 2 credits can be claimed by preceptors. Medical school and residency program administrators can send letters confirming and documenting your participation.

CME Discounts

Participating in an institution's community-based teaching program may qualify the preceptor for discounts on CME programs, including conferences and printed, electronic, and Web-based products. Some programs may be willing to audiotape their grand rounds and make them available at no charge so preceptors can earn CME credit when it is more convenient to participate.

Internet and E-mail

Many programs have the capability to connect their community-based office practices to the Internet, thus allowing the preceptor and learner access to literature-retrieval databases (e.g., MEDLINE), e-mail, the institution's health care database, and teaching resources. As a further incentive, tutorials on how to use these various programs and services can be provided by the sponsoring institution.

Textbooks

Textbooks can be provided to some office sites by the sponsoring institution.

Faculty-Development Programs

Some institutions offer faculty-development programs for their preceptors. National programs are also available, and the ACP-ASIM Community-Based Teaching Program loans and sells faculty-development videos and companion texts to improve the teaching skills of preceptors. Community-based teaching faculty development can also be offered at regional ACP-ASIM meetings. Contact the ACP-ASIM Community-Based Teaching Program via the Internet for the latest information on national faculty-development programs or its videos at http://www.acponline.org/cme/cbt or call 800-523-1546, ext. 2588.

Recognition Dinners

Annual receptions or dinners recognize the volunteer efforts of the preceptors are a popular method of distributing preceptor awards. These events can be used to hand out either teaching awards or recognition certificates.

Certificates of Appreciation

Most local programs offer certificates or letters of appreciation. ACP-ASIM offers two national awards: the Community-Based Teaching Participation Award and the Community-Based Teaching Excellence in Teaching Award (see ACP-ASIM Awards Program in Appendix C). For more information call 800-523-1546, ext. 2588.

Index